M000277187

Wartarin

and the effects of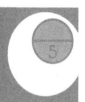

Vitamin K

+ Protein

includes tables of Vitamin K and
Protein content in common foods

Cath Atkin

ISBN: 978-0-9933499-1-1

Copyright © 2016 Cath Atkin

www.eatonwarfarin.com

Disclaimer

This book is not designed, or intended, to provide you with medical advice, professional diagnosis, opinion, treatment or services. This book is not intended as a substitute for the medical advice of doctors or other medical or healthcare professionals. You should regularly consult a doctor (or other relevant medical professional) in matters relating to your health. You should not use the information in this book as a substitute for a consultation with a doctor or other medical professional.

Although the author has made every effort to ensure that the information in this book was correct at the time of publication, the author and the publisher do not assume and hereby disclaim any liability to any party for any loss, damage, or disruption caused by errors or omissions, whether such errors or omissions result from negligence, accident, or any other cause. The author is not liable or responsible for any advice, course of treatment, diagnosis or any other information or services you obtain or follow as a result of reading this book.

IF YOU BELIEVE YOU HAVE A MEDICAL EMERGENCY, YOU SHOULD IMMEDIATELY CALL THE RELEVANT EMERGENCY SERVICES IN YOUR JURISDICTION. If you believe you have any other health problem, or if you have any questions regarding your health, you should promptly consult your doctor (or other relevant healthcare professionals). Never disregard medical or professional advice, or delay seeking it on account of something you read in this book. Do not rely on information in this book instead of seeking professional medical advice. You should also ask your physician, or other healthcare professionals, to assist you in interpreting the information in this book or in applying this information to your individual case.

Medical information changes constantly. Therefore the information in this book should not be considered current, complete or exhaustive, nor should you rely on such information to recommend a course of treatment for you or any other individual.

Acknowledgements

Special thanks and gratitude to my colleague, Laura Draper, for all her hard work, diligence and patience!

We hope this book and website will make a positive difference to those on Warfarin…

…wishing you well.

CONTENTS

For further information and resources
visit
www.eatonwarfarin.com

Introduction

Following on from writing my first book, *Warfarin: An easy to follow guide from a patient's perspective* I decided to take a more in-depth look at some of the dietary considerations for Warfarin users.

In the earlier book I touched on the importance of having consistent amounts of Vitamin K in your diet. Personal experience has highlighted to me that it is also important to watch the amount of protein you consume when taking Warfarin.

In this book I go into a lot more detail about the significance of monitoring both Vitamin K and protein intake when on Warfarin. As before, I have tried to keep explanations simple and make this a straightforward guide with quick access to the important facts. I hope you will find this useful.

About the Author

*At the age of just 41 my world fell apart when, completely out of the blue, I suffered a **stroke**. Further tests revealed that the cause of this unexpected event was a blood clotting disorder called <u>antiphospholipid syndrome</u> **(APS)**. As a result of this diagnosis of APS, which is also known as **Hughes syndrome**, I was prescribed **Warfarin** immediately and told that I would be on it for the rest of my life.*

*In trying to work out what this was going to mean for me I discovered it was hard to find straightforward, **easy to understand** information about Warfarin, and this led me to write my first book. My aim was to provide a <u>simple and quick to read guide</u> for anyone coming into contact with Warfarin, particularly those who have been newly prescribed it, or are supporting someone who has to take it. It also <u>tells of my journey</u> from the circumstances that led to my stroke, through to how I coped with the various aspects of being on Warfarin and **learning to <u>balance</u> my <u>diet</u> and <u>warfarin therapy</u>.***

*... and so to the next leg of my journey as a '**Warfarinite**', because that is exactly what being on Warfarin has been for me ..... a journey. Just when I think I am getting to grips with everything, some new problem or setback comes along and needs resolved – but I just accept this as **part of the process** and work through it to find an answer.*

So, what can I eat on Warfarin?

*Maintaining a **healthy diet** has always played an important part in my life but since being on Warfarin I have struggled with **interactions** between my **diet** and my warfarin therapy and I have found **losing weight a particular challenge**. I love salads - I used to live on them in the summer – but because I was trying to be careful about the amount of Vitamin K in my diet while taking Warfarin I started eating other things. It wasn't long before I realised that I was putting on more and more weight. You know what it is like – before you know it you have gone up yet another clothes size!*

*I decided that enough was enough. I had to do something about it so I started to look around for a **diet** that I wouldn't mind doing (well there is no point in me starting a diet that I don't enjoy or I just won't stick to it!). There are so many diets out there nowadays that you would think it was just a case of picking one.....*

*Well, **when you are on Warfarin, it is not quite that easy!** A large number of diets and healthy eating plans contain very high levels of Vitamin K. You only have to google 'weight loss' or 'healthy eating' to be inundated with images of green shakes or broccoli! In the past I would have been all for a 'green' diet but now I can only eat this type of food in moderation.*

The diet I decided on was based around 'Clean Eating' *which is about <u>avoiding processed and refined foods and</u>* <u>*eating only 'whole' foods*</u>*. I also reduced my* **gluten** *intake* *significantly (as this apparently helps the* **auto immune** **disorder** *that I have) and continued to be careful of my* *Vitamin K intake. I thought, why not deal with two things* *at once – losing weight and also improving the health of* *my immune system? I knew that I was eating healthily, and* *was soon rewarded with some weight loss, so I couldn't* *understand why I <u>started to feel ill</u>? Things got progres-* *sively worse so I eventually made an appointment to have* *my INR checked. I was shocked by the results that came* *back -* ***my INR was drastically low!***

I went back and checked the ***food diary*** *I had been keeping* *to see if I could make sense of this. At first I wondered if* *the amount of Potassium in my diet was having an effect* *on my Warfarin but I could find no research to support this.* *What I did find, however, was that as a result of reducing* *sugars and refined carbohydrates in my diet, and limiting* *the amount of vegetables I was eating, I was* ***consuming*** ***substantially more <u>protein</u> than normal.***

Further investigation revealed that ***<u>high protein levels</u>*** ***<u>can significantly decrease INR</u>*** *– something I had* *been completely unaware of!*

*Once again I felt the frustration of not having enough guidance or information to make the right choices about my eating.   I was determined to find the answers and come up with a <u>healthy eating regime</u> that would allow me to **lose weight, balance** my **Vitamin K and protein** levels and keep my **INR stable** whilst also addressing other health issues through diet (in my case auto immune and thyroid).*

The results of my research are contained in this book. I hope I can help others avoid the pitfalls I encountered and find strategies to eat healthily, and lose weight if required, while taking Warfarin.

CHAPTER 1

*Warfarin –
The Basics*

The purpose of this book is not to explain how Warfarin works, however, this chapter provides a quick recap of the things you should know if you want to fully understand how to manage your Warfarin therapy.

Coagulation, or **clotting of the blood**, is what stops us bleeding to death if we are cut or injured. Good news on the whole, but *some people are at risk of blood clots forming too easily* and this can lead to serious health events such as **heart attack, stroke, pulmonary embolism (PE) or deep vein thrombosis (DVT).**

Warfarin is one of a number of medications that can be prescribed to **help prevent these unwanted blood clots forming.** In simple terms, it does this by interfering with the clotting process as follows,

Clotting of the blood is controlled by a group of **proteins** made in the liver called **clotting factors**. For these proteins to function they **need a supply of** Vitamin K.

Warfarin works by,

1. <u>Reducing</u> the production of **proteins** in the liver

2. <u>Limiting</u> the availability of **Vitamin K**

and, as a result, it takes longer for the blood to clot and unwanted blood clots are less likely to form.

While Warfarin's ability to prevent blood clots <u>saves many lives</u>, there is a flip side to this. Because Warfarin slows down the clotting of the blood, <u>too high a dose</u> could cause **life-threatening bleeding**.

It is, therefore, vital that your dosage is monitored so that your health professional can prescribe <u>the correct level of Warfarin for you</u>. This is achieved by regular blood tests.

Your doctor will frequently carry out a <u>Prothrombin time test</u> which is the name of the blood test used to measure the time it takes for your blood to clot. This is then reported as a number known as your **INR** (<u>International Normalised Ratio</u>).

It is important to become familiar with the term **INR**, and to understand the part this number plays in the management of your Warfarin levels. In simple terms,

If the **INR is too low** - blood clots cannot be prevented

If the **INR is too high** - there is an increased risk of bleeding

Your doctor, or anticoagulant specialist, will decide on the correct **INR** for you and will aim to keep it within a desired range.   This is known as your Therapeutic Range.

*Although Warfarin has been widely used as an anti-coagulant for over 60 years, in my experience there is still a great deal of negativity towards it.   Originally developed as a rat poison, this is a label that Warfarin has struggled to shake off.   However, it is now responsible for keeping me, and many hundreds of thousands like me, safer by reducing the likelihood of fatal blood clots developing. I, for one, welcome it. Being on Warfarin has required me to make **changes to my lifestyle**.   The key is all about **balance**, being **consistent** and not making sudden or major changes. Not a very exciting way to live you might think!   But when you compare it to getting very unwell or being at risk of another clotting event, it is a price worth* *paying in my mind. Yes, it can sometimes be a pain having to keep getting my bloods checked and watching my diet but the more I have looked into how food, drink and other factors can affect Warfarin therapy the more success I am experiencing in managing to have **a balanced diet <u>and</u> stable INR**. Ultimately I would like to be able to reduce my Warfarin intake and continue to maintain a stable INR just by eating and drinking a carefully managed diet (and without putting myself at risk) but, as I said, it is a journey ....*

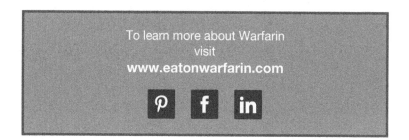

To learn more about Warfarin
visit
www.eatonwarfarin.com

CHAPTER 2

BloodWATCH System

In my first book I introduced a system called <u>BloodWATCH</u>.

I came up with this system because I found most of the **terminology** used to explain about Warfarin, and its interactions with other things, *more than a little confusing!*

I just <u>wanted to be able to tell at a glance</u> if something could put me **at risk of either bleeding or clotting**!

I felt sure that I would not be alone in this so I created a unique system called <u>BloodWATCH</u> which provides a **quick key** to the **potential risks** for Warfarin users of any factors being discussed.

Anything which can put you at **increased risk of bleeding** will be denoted by *this text* or the following symbol:

Anything which can put you at **increased risk of clotting** will be denoted by **this text** or the following symbol:

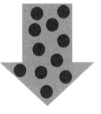

You will find this same system in use in all my books, and on our website www.eatonwarfarin.com, so whatever you are reading about you will easily be able to identify any associated risks.

To link the BloodWATCH System with the other terminology used in this book I have put together a table which you can use as a quick reference. This should also assist you to interpret what you read about Warfarin elsewhere.

Increase in **anticoagulant effect**	Increased risk of bleeding	
Decrease in **anticoagulant effect**	Increased risk of clotting	
Increase in **'blood thinning'**	Increased risk of bleeding	
Decrease in **'blood thinning'**	Increased risk of clotting	
Increase in **clotting rate**	Increased risk of clotting	
Decrease in **clotting rate**	Increased risk of bleeding	
INR **below** Therapeutic Range	Increased risk of clotting	
INR **above** Therapeutic Range	Increased risk of bleeding	
Increase in **effect of Warfarin**	Increased risk of bleeding	
Decrease in **effect of Warfarin**	Increased risk of clotting	
Increasing **INR**	Increased risk of bleeding	
Decreasing **INR**	Increased risk of clotting	
Reduced platelet function	Increased risk of bleeding	

For more information on **BloodWATCH** or to download a copy of
this table visit **www.eatonwarfarin.com**

CHAPTER 3

Vitamin K and Warfarin: what you need to know

*Having always enjoyed a healthy diet of salads and vegetables, with spinach and broccoli being among my favourites, it came as a bit of a blow to discover that as a Warfarin user I was going to have to <u>limit the amount of Vitamin K</u> I ate. I am writing this in early January – a time when so many people are turning their thoughts to finding healthy eating regimes to help them get over the excesses of the holiday season. Everywhere you look there are new **diets** popping up and doctors and health professionals extolling the virtues of **green leafy vegetables** and other **Vitamin K** laden delicacies! It's torture!!! But seriously, as you will discover below <u>being on Warfarin **doesn't** mean avoiding Vitamin K completely.</u> In fact it is really important that you **DO** include sufficient Vitamin K in your diet!*

When you are prescribed Warfarin one of the first things that is highlighted to you is the **significant effect that Vitamin K can have on your INR.**

To recap,

An **increased amount of Vitamin K** can **lower your INR** making Warfarin less effective and potentially increasing the <u>risk of blood clots</u>.

A *decreased amount of Vitamin K* can **increase your INR** making Warfarin more effective and putting you at <u>risk of bleeding</u>.

<u>This does not mean that you must avoid Vitamin K but rather that the amount of Vitamin K you have in your diet should be</u> **consistent**.

The guidance on **Vitamin K intake** can be a bit bewildering and it is easy to understand why Warfarin patients may think they should substantially reduce the amount of Vitamin K they consume, or even leave it out of their diet altogether!   However, this <u>can lead to Vitamin K deficiency</u> which has many health implications.

Vitamin K is an **essential nutrient** and, as well as being **vital** in allowing our blood to clot, research suggests that it provides **other important health benefits,**

- *Protecting against heart disease* by inhibiting calcification of the arteries

- Improving bone density thus *reducing the risk of fractures and osteoporosis*

- Possibly contributing towards the *prevention of cancers and dementia*

Perhaps even more importantly for Warfarin users, it has been shown that **regularly consuming a moderate amount of Vitamin K** actually <u>**helps to achieve a more consistent and stable INR!**</u>

It is **essential**, therefore, not only to eat <u>*consistent amounts of Vitamin K*</u> but also to ensure that this <u>*daily amount is adequate.*</u>

How much Vitamin K should you include in your diet?

In the UK, the NHS recommends that the <u>**minimum**</u> daily intake of Vitamin K for an average <u>man</u> is **90 micrograms (µg)** and for an average <u>woman</u> is **75 micrograms (µg)**. Other countries may differ, for example, in Canada and the US the minimum recommended daily amounts are 120 µg for men and 90 µg for women.

The exact daily amount you decide to include in

your diet is not too critical because as long as you maintain roughly the same intake of Vitamin K each day then your Warfarin dosage can be adjusted by your doctor to reflect this.

You should, however, **discuss with your doctor** before making any big changes in the amount of Vitamin K in your daily diet so that your **INR can be closely monitored**.

Sources of Vitamin K

There are 2 types of Vitamin K found in food – **Vitamin K₁** and **Vitamin K₂**.

Vitamin K₁

Vitamin K₁ (also known as **phylloquinone**) is **produced by plants** and is the main dietary source of Vitamin K. There are 3 main food groups that contain significant amounts of Vitamin K₁.

Vegetables, particularly dark green leafy vegetables such as spinach or kale, are where the largest quantities of Vitamin K₁ are found. *As a general rule*, **the greener and leafier the vegetable,**

the more Vitamin K it will contain!

<u>Oils</u> are the next **major source of Vitamin K**$_1$ although this varies greatly depending on the type of oil;

- **rapeseed, soya** and **olive oil** are all <u>**high** in</u> <u>Vitamin K</u>

- **sunflower, corn** and **coconut oil**, contain only <u>**small** amounts of Vitamin K</u>.

As well as containing Vitamin K, it has been suggested that **fats and oils increase the absorption of Vitamin K in foods.**

<u>**Processed foods**</u>, particularly <u>fast foods</u> and <u>snacks</u>, are the third category of foods where **considerable amounts of Vitamin K**$_1$ have been found. This is because oils such as rapeseed and soya oil are used in their production, or sometimes they are just **cooked in oils** which are <u>high in</u> <u>Vitamin K</u>. Foods that are commonly produced, or cooked, using high Vitamin K containing oils include **burgers, French fries, corn snacks, crisps, cakes** and **salad dressings**. It should be noted, however, that this varies greatly from one brand to another depending on the actual oils and quantities used.

Many processed foods also contain a hydrogenated form of Vitamin K_1 known as dihydrophylloquinone (dK). However, this dK is much less well absorbed and so does not impact on Vitamin K status in the same way as Vitamin K_1.

Most other foods contain only small, or trace, amounts of Vitamin K_1. One other thing to watch out for is produce that has an **'added' Vitamin K content**. Typically, <u>nutritional supplements</u>, <u>energy bars</u> and <u>diet shakes</u> will have **Vitamin K added** and could contain, for example, around **20 micrograms in one bar!**

Vitamin K_2

Vitamin K_2 (also known as **menaquinone**) is **formed in nature from bacteria**. A small amount of Vitamin K_2 *occurs naturally in the body* where it is synthesised by bacteria in the intestine. Otherwise, Vitamin K_2 is present in a <u>limited number of foodstuffs</u> but it is **not a major dietary source of Vitamin K**.

Foods containing **Vitamin K_2** in <u>**significant amounts**</u> include **eggs, fermented foods** and **some cheeses**. It may also be found to a lesser extent in **cow liver** and **chicken.**

The best known source of Vitamin K_2 is a foodstuff called **natto**. This is a dish containing **fermented soybeans** which is eaten in parts of Japan. It has been attributed to low rates of heart disease and osteoporosis in Japan but its' somewhat 'unusual' flavour means it may be unlikely to be adopted by the rest of the world any time soon! Recently, however, natto has been mentioned in a number of articles about 'superfoods'.

Special Considerations for Babies and Children

It can be particularly tricky to regulate the intake of Vitamin K in a child's diet. For babies and children being treated with Warfarin there are a number of factors which can significantly influence their Vitamin K levels and these must be taken into account when managing their warfarin therapy.

For **babies** at the **milk feeding stage**, the way in which they are being fed will have an effect on the amount of Vitamin K they are getting. **Breast milk does not contain large amounts of Vitamin K.** *Infant formula*, on the other hand, *is enriched with Vitamin K* so bottle fed babies are likely to take in more Vitamin K than their breast fed counterparts. Similarly, some babies and children on Warfarin may have **conditions** which require them to obtain their nutrition by a route which *bypasses the normal process of drinking and eating.* **Feeds which are tube fed directly into the stomach, or vein**, should have a carefully calculated amount of Vitamin K contained in the nutritional mixture. However, possible inconsistencies mean that children who need these methods of feeding whilst on warfarin will have **both their feed and their INR carefully monitored.**

*I am often asked if breast feeding is safe for a baby whose mother is on Warfarin. I have not experienced this myself but all the research out there points to warfarin being safe in lactation as it does not pass into the breast milk in any **detectible amounts**. If you are in any doubt about whether breast feeding is safe for you, and your baby, check with your Doctor, Midwife or Health Visitor.*

For older children eating and digesting food normally, parents should be mindful of the high amounts of **Vitamin K** contained in some **fast foods** and **snacks**. While vegetables such as broccoli and cabbage contain large quantities of Vitamin K, many children (particularly 'fussy eaters') are more likely to get their Vitamin K intake from foods that have been <u>cooked in Vitamin K rich oils</u>. Foods such as **chips, burgers, French fries, crisps** and **corn snacks** are very often cooked in rapeseed and vegetable oils making them an <u>unexpected</u> source of Vitamin K. Whatever, the source of Vitamin K, the **key for parents** is to **keep their child's diet as consistent as possible to maintain a stable INR.**

The health problems that require children to be prescribed warfarin, **predominately heart conditions**, will in themselves present a number of complications in achieving consistency of Vitamin K intake. Many of these children will have gut conditions that will <u>affect the absorption of nutrients such as Vitamin K</u>. They are also more likely to be prone to infections and illnesses, leading to sickness and diarrhoea, **which can quickly upset the Vitamin K levels** in the body and **put the child at risk of bleeding**.

Nutritional Data for Vitamin K

As it is important for Warfarin users to <u>monitor</u> the amount of Vitamin K they are consuming, *access to reliable data on the Vitamin K content of foods is essential.*

Testing of foodstuffs to determine the Vitamin K content has, unfortunately, not been given a lot of focus over the years. There are a number of reasons why this has been the case. It has only been in fairly recent times that the ***health benefits of Vitamin K*** have become more fully recognised and, to date, the requirement for information on Vitamin K values has not been driven by regulation. The difficult processes involved in analysing foods to measure Vitamin K content, coupled with a lack of commercial demand for this information, has also led to research in this area being limited.

The research that is available has, wherever possible, been based on taking an average from a number of different samples. This is important because it has been shown that the amount of Vitamin K found in some foodstuffs can vary depending on a range of factors.

In **vegetables**, the growing conditions, soil type and climate have been shown to have an impact on the amount of Vitamin K they contain. Similarly, the age of the plant will affect the values reported.

Even, the part of the plant that the sample is taken from is significant **e.g. the inner and outer leaves of a cabbage will contain different amounts of Vitamin K.**

Interestingly, research suggests that cooking and freezing have little, or no effect, on the Vitamin K content of vegetables. This is believed to be because Vitamin K is fat soluble, rather than water soluble.

When comparing raw and cooked vegetables, you may notice that very often the Vitamin K **content for cooked vegetables is higher** than that of the same vegetable in its' **raw state**. This difference is to do with vegetables, like spinach, cooking down and resulting in a more concentrated form rather than cooking increasing the amount of Vitamin K present.

With **oils**, the Vitamin K content can be affected by storage conditions. Exposure to heat and light have both been shown to reduce the amount of Vitamin K contained within oils.

In the case of **processed foods**, you would expect to find small variations in the precise amount of Vitamin K contained in different batches of the same product. **Different brands can also vary**

significantly. Unfortunately, not many food manufacturers provide Vitamin K values for their products. However, by checking the **type and percentage of oils listed in the ingredients** it is possible to get a guide to whether the product is likely to be high in Vitamin K.

Despite the limitations and possible variations discussed above, the data contained in the Vitamin K tables in **Chapter 5** should be comprehensive enough to enable the user to *track their Vitamin K* intake with sufficient accuracy. These tables contain a wide range of commonly consumed foods arranged in 3 different formats.

CHAPTER 4

Protein and Warfarin: what you need to know

An attempt to **get healthy** and **lose some weight** left me feeling extremely unwell and led me to the discovery that **having too much protein in the diet** <u>should be avoided</u> by anyone taking Warfarin. What I thought was a very 'healthy' diet actually **caused a dramatic decrease in my INR** which, apart from making me ill, put me at <u>**greater risk of having a clot**</u>. I was following a **'clean eating'** approach, which meant I tried not to eat anything **processed** or **pasteurised**, instead eating more fresh foods (all the while being mindful of my Vitamin K intake!). I was also trying to eliminate gluten (proteins found in wheat and other grains) from my diet as this <u>exacerbates an auto immune disorder</u> that I have. Not a lot to concentrate on then!

As a result I was eating far less sugars, refined carbohydrates and processed foods. Instead my diet consisted of **'whole' foods** such as **meat, fish, nuts** and **eggs**. I followed recipes that replaced wheat flour with almond flour (ground almonds). My favourite breakfast was nut granola, using almond milk instead of cow's milk, topped with a whole banana and a little almond butter to top up my healthy fats for the day. Sounds good? Sounds healthy? Well it is, but *just not for someone who needs to maintain a stable INR! What I had done, without realising, was to* **hugely _increase_ the amount of _protein_ I was consuming** which was, in turn, steadily **_decreasing my INR to critical levels._**

When you are first prescribed Warfarin you will be told about certain things to watch out for such as being consistent with your Vitamin K intake and avoiding cranberry juice. There are many more things, which you won't necessarily be told about, that can affect the stability of your INR. **One of these is Protein.**

How Protein affects Warfarin

A number of studies have been undertaken to look at the effect of protein on Warfarin. In several documented cases it has been shown that there is a **significant link** between high protein intake and a decrease in INR.

While the exact mechanism for this is not known, it is thought that this is connected to the level of protein in the bloodstream.

Basically, when you take Warfarin some of it **attaches** itself to **albumin**, which is the main **protein in human blood**. Any Warfarin that does stick to the albumin in your bloodstream will then **not be available to perform its role as an anticoagulant**. It would therefore follow that if consuming a lot of *protein* *increases* the amount of *albumin in your bloodstream* then *more* of your *Warfarin will become attached to it*. **This all results in less of your Warfarin being available to do its 'blood thinning' job.**

There are a number of other factors that could explain why being on a high protein diet, such as the Atkins Diet or a Paleo approach, could bring about a decrease in INR. Generally, when someone is following this type of diet they will consume a lot more fat and, as we discussed in the Vitamin K chapter, **fats and oils can enhance the absorption of Vitamin K**. Also, as these diets tend to limit carbohydrates this will often result in more vegetables being eaten which could potentially **increase Vitamin K intake**.

How much Protein should you include in your diet?

Protein is incredibly important to the human body. It is one of the body's main building blocks and is **essential for growth, repair** and **maintaining good health.** Clearly we need to include protein in our diets but how much protein do we actually need to keep us healthy?

Dietary Reference Values (DRVs) provide the UK population with a guide to what is a sufficient daily intake of a particular nutrient. For protein, the recommended **DRV is 0.75g per kilogram of body weight** which amounts to,

> **55g**   **per day** for the average **man**
>
> **45g**   **per day** for the average **woman**

Most people easily exceed this target with the current average daily protein intake in the UK being,

> **88g**   per day for **men**
>
> **64g**   per day for **women**

The advice given by the **UK Department of Health** is that **adults <u>should not</u> eat more than double the recommended intake of protein each day**.

Excessive protein has been linked with, among other things, kidney problems and issues with bone health.

For Warfarin users, a more moderate approach of **aiming** to eat around the guideline <u>recommended daily intake is probably advisable</u>.

Sources of Protein

Protein is found in varying quantities in the following food types,

Meat – such as beef, pork and lamb

Poultry – such as chicken and turkey

Fish – such as haddock, tuna and lobster

Eggs and **Dairy** – such as chicken eggs, milk and cheese

Nuts and **Seeds** – such as almonds, peanuts and sunflower seeds

Pulses – such as kidney beans, lentils and split peas

Cereals and **Grains** – such as quinoa

Soy Products – such as tofu

Fruits – such as banana and avocado

Nutritional Data for Protein

It is relatively easy to monitor the amount of protein you are consuming as information on the protein content of foods is readily available. Wherever nutritional information is given on food packaging, the amount of protein will always be included as it is one of **the 'Big 4' nutrients** that are listed as a minimum.

The demand for complete and reliable food composition data has led to the development of a wide range of highly sensitive and accurate methods of detecting the concentration of protein in food materials.

Chapter 5 contains tables of data on the protein content of commonly consumed foods.

CHAPTER 5

*Vitamin K
and Protein
Tables*

The tables in this book draw on some of the most up to date sources of nutritional data available. Arranged in two different formats, these tables are designed to assist with meal planning and recording your daily intake of Vitamin K and protein.

Table 1: Vitamin K – High to Low – a direct comparison of the <u>amount</u> of Vitamin K found <u>in 100g</u> of a selected range of foods.

Table 2: Protein – High to Low – a direct comparison of the <u>amount</u> of Protein found <u>in 100g</u> of a selected range of foods.

Table 3: Vitamin K and Protein – A to Z – a table of commonly consumed foods (arranged alphabetically) providing the Vitamin K and protein <u>content</u> of <u>a standard serving</u>.

Please note:-

The nutritional contents given in these tables represent average values. The reliability of all food data is subject to the natural variations in foods and should be used as a guide only.

Table 1: **Vitamin K – High to Low**

	Vitamin K$_1$ μg per 100g	Vitamin K$_2$ μg per 100g
Basil, dried, ground	1714.50	
Sage, dried, ground	1714.50	
Thyme, dried, ground	1714.50	
Parsley, dried	1359.50	
Coriander leaves, dried	1359.50	
Amaranth leaves, raw	1140.00	
Spring greens, boiled	893.00	
Kale, frozen, boiled	882.00	
Spinach, frozen, boiled	840.00	
Swiss Chard, raw	830.00	
Kale, fresh, boiled	817.00	
Dandelion greens, raw	778.40	
Kale, raw	623.00	
Oregano, dried, ground	621.70	
Marjoram, dried	621.70	
Mustard greens (leaves), fresh, boiled	592.70	
Spinach, fresh, boiled	575.00	
Dandelion greens, fresh, boiled	551.40	
Parsley, fresh	548.00	
Garden cress, raw	541.90	
Nettles, blanched	498.60	
Beet greens, fresh, boiled	484.00	
Basil, fresh	414.80	
Collards, fresh, boiled	406.60	
Beet greens, raw	400.00	
Spinach, raw	394.00	
Mustard greens (leaves), frozen, boiled	335.10	
Swiss Chard, fresh, boiled	327.30	
Watercress, raw	315.00	
Coriander leaves, fresh	310.00	

	Vitamin K$_1$ µg per 100g	Vitamin K$_2$ µg per 100g
Bhaji, spinach and potato, homemade	284.45	
Mustard greens (leaves), raw	257.50	
Raddiccio, raw	255.20	
Green cabbage, raw	242.00	
Endive, raw	231.00	
Chives, fresh	212.70	
Spring onions, bulbs and tops, raw	207.00	
Green cabbage, fresh, boiled	201.00	
Broccoli, raw	185.00	
Soybean oil	183.90	
Black pepper	163.70	
Mayonnaise, standard retail	163.00	
Brussels sprouts, fresh, raw	153.00	
Cloves, ground	141.80	
Broccoli, fresh, boiled	135.00	
Soya oil	131.00	
Lettuce, average, raw	129.00	
Brussels sprouts, fresh, boiled	127.00	
High Protein Shake, powder only	125.00	
Brussels sprouts, frozen, boiled	119.50	
Rapeseed oil (Canola)	112.50	
Vegetable oil	112.50	
Rocket, raw (Arugula)	108.60	
Taro leaves, raw	108.60	
Chilli powder	105.70	
Cos lettuce, raw	102.50	
Romaine lettuce, raw	102.50	
Curry powder	99.80	
SLIMFAST Shake powder	96.20	
Broccoli, frozen, boiled	88.10	
Mustard cress, raw	88.00	
Broccoli, frozen, unprepared	81.10	
Paprika, ground	80.30	

	Vitamin K_1 µg per 100g	Vitamin K_2 µg per 100g
Cayenne pepper, ground	80.30	
Asparagus, frozen, boiled	80.00	
Vegetable pakora, retail	72.10	
COMPLAN powder	67.00	
Kelp, raw	66.00	
Fennel bulb, raw	62.80	
White cabbage, raw	60.00	
Prunes, dried	59.50	
Olive oil	57.50	
Pine nut kernels	53.90	
Mayonnaise, reduced fat	53.70	
Asparagus, fresh, boiled	51.82	
Okra, frozen, boiled	47.80	
Red cabbage, boiled	47.60	
Pak Choi, raw	45.50	
Asparagus, raw	41.60	
White cabbage, fresh, boiled	41.21	
Celeriac, raw	41.00	
Fava beans, raw	40.90	
Kiwi fruit, raw	40.30	
Okra, boiled	40.00	
Green beans, raw	39.00	
Peas, fresh, boiled	39.00	
Peas, raw	39.00	
Red cabbage, raw	38.20	
Cashew nuts, roasted	34.70	
Pak choi, steamed	34.00	
Beansprouts, mung, raw	33.00	
Cauliflower bhaji, homemade	32.70	
Okra, raw	31.30	
Cinnamon, ground	31.20	
Cauliflower, raw	31.00	
Alfalfa sprouts, raw	30.50	

	Vitamin K₁ µg per 100g	Vitamin K₂ µg per 100g
Peas, canned	30.40	
Miso	29.30	
Rhubarb stems, raw	29.30	
Cauliflower, fresh, boiled	28.50	
Peas, frozen, raw	27.90	0
Prunes, stewed	26.10	
Runner beans	26.00	
Spirulina, dried	25.50	
Soya flour	25.30	
Cocoa butter	24.70	
Soybean oil (partially hydrongenated)	24.70	
Beef dripping	24.50	
Iceberg lettuce	24.10	
Peas, frozen, boiled	24.00	
Natto	23.10	
Mushy peas, canned	22.50	
Avocado, raw	21.00	
Tortilla chips, fried in sunflower oil	20.90	
Cucumber, raw	20.90	
Blackberries, raw	19.80	
BURGER KING WHOPPER (no cheese)	19.50	
Blueberries, raw	19.30	
Jalapeno peppers	18.50	
Carrots, frozen, unprepared	17.60	
Pomegranate	16.40	
Puff pastry, frozen, ready-to-bake	16.10	
McDONALDS FRENCH FRIES	16.00	
Figs, dried	15.60	
Corn snacks e.g. WOTSITS	15.50	
Mangetout, fresh, boiled	15.00	
Walnut oil	15.00	
Globe artichoke, boiled	14.80	
Grapes, red + green	14.60	

	Vitamin K$_1$ µg per 100g	Vitamin K$_2$ µg per 100g
Split peas, dried, raw	14.50	
Chilli pepper, green, raw	14.30	
Hazelnuts	14.20	
Chilli pepper, red, raw	14.00	
Cooking fat	13.80	
Carrots, frozen, boiled	13.60	
Sesame oil	13.60	
Turmeric, ground	13.40	
Pistachio nuts, roasted	13.20	
Tomatoes, grilled	12.50	
Broad beans, frozen, boiled	11.40	
Bran, wheat	10.40	
Leeks, raw	10.10	
Potato snacks e.g. PRINGLES	9.60	
Leeks, fresh, boiled	9.50	
Flaxseed oil	9.30	0
Carrots, young	9.20	
Chick peas, raw	8.92	
Gram flour	8.92	
Dark chocolate, 45-59% cacao solids	8.10	0.1
Palm oil	7.90	
Green beans, frozen, boiled	7.80	
Raspberries	7.80	
Roasted chestnuts	7.80	
Plums	7.50	
Butter	7.40	
Dark chocolate, 70-85% cacao solids	7.30	0
Beef mince, stewed	7.18	
Almond oil	7.00	
SLIMFAST Shake, ready to drink	6.50	
Double cream, fresh	6.40	
Green pepper	6.40	
Sunflower oil	6.30	

	Vitamin K_1 µg per 100g	Vitamin K_2 µg per 100g
Aubergine	6.10	
COFFEEMATE, whitener	6.00	
Tomatoes	6.00	
Rye flour	5.90	
Peaches	5.80	
Apples, average	5.60	
Dates	5.60	
Carrots, old	5.50	
Mustard seeds	5.40	
Cumin seeds	5.40	
Cranberries	5.10	
Goose, meat, fat + skin, roasted	5.10	
Lentils, green and brown, dried	5.00	
Pheasant, roasted	4.90	
Celery, raw	4.90	
Fennel, fresh, boiled	4.90	
MARS bar	4.80	
Cheddar cheese	4.70	8.6
Full fat soft cheese	4.70	
Lamb, shoulder, lean + fat, roasted	4.60	
Lamb, stewing, lean, braised	4.40	
Winter squash	4.40	
Flaxseeds	4.30	
Instant coffee powder	4.30	
Quail	4.20	
Red kidney beans, canned	4.10	
Danish blue cheese	4.10	
Duck, meat only, roasted	3.80	
Biscuits, cream sandwich e.g. Custard Creams	3.80	
Cranberries, dried, sweetened	3.80	
Dried onions	3.80	
Naan bread, retail	3.80	
Raisins	3.70	

	Vitamin K_1 µg per 100g	Vitamin K_2 µg per 100g
Beef suet	3.60	
Lamb, mince, raw	3.60	
Pears	3.60	
Pecan nuts	3.50	
Chocolate biscuit e.g. BREAKAWAY	3.46	
Ostrich, top loin, cooked	3.40	
Safflower oil	3.40	
Tomato puree	3.40	
Apricots	3.30	
Courgette	3.30	
Oat bran	3.20	
Beef, liver	3.10	
Corn oil	3.00	
Goat's cheese, hard	3.00	
Houmous	3.00	
Strawberries	3.00	
Honeydew melon	2.90	
Potatoes, red, flesh + skin	2.90	
Beef, mince, raw	2.90	
Pretzels	2.80	
Duck, meat only, raw	2.80	
Dates, deglet noor + medjool	2.70	
Gruyere cheese	2.70	
Walnuts	2.70	
Fontina cheese	2.60	
Guava	2.60	
Papaya	2.60	
Sardines, canned in oil, drained	2.60	
Canteloupe melon	2.50	
Mozzarella cheese	2.50	
Swiss cheese	2.50	
Beef, braising steak, lean + fat	2.50	
Goat's cheese, semisoft	2.50	

	Vitamin K$_1$ µg per 100g	Vitamin K$_2$ µg per 100g
Monterey cheese	2.50	
Nectarines	2.50	
Peaches, canned in syrup	2.40	
Blue cheese	2.40	
Brie	2.40	
Marrow	2.40	
Port Salut cheese	2.40	
Tofu, soya bean	2.40	
Sweet potato, baked	2.30	
Edam cheese	2.30	
Gouda cheese	2.30	
Plain chocolate, 36-50% cocoa solids	2.30	
Tomato juice	2.30	
Yam	2.30	
Chick peas, dried, boiled	2.24	
Apricots, canned	2.20	
Pearl barley, raw	2.20	
Provolone cheese	2.20	
Romano cheese	2.20	
Strawberries	2.20	
Sweet potato, boiled	2.10	
Cherries	2.10	
Camembert cheese	2.00	
Corned beef	2.00	
Pumpkin flesh, boiled	2.00	
Swede	2.00	
Wholemeal bread	2.00	
Beef, brisket, lean+ fat, boiled	1.90	
Beef, sirloin steak, lean + fat, raw	1.90	
Cassava	1.90	
Chocolate nut spread	1.90	
Wheat flour, whole-grain	1.90	
Wild rice	1.90	

	Vitamin K_1 µg per 100g	Vitamin K_2 µg per 100g
Sour cream	1.80	
Sweet potato, raw	1.80	
Feta cheese	1.80	
Goat's cheese, soft	1.80	
Biscuits, semi-sweet e.g. Rich Tea	1.71	
Soymilk	1.71	
Parmesan, grated	1.70	7.1
Garlic	1.70	
Chorizo	1.60	
Ginger nut biscuits	1.60	
Processed Cheese	1.60	
Red peppers	1.60	
Cheese, average hard	1.57	
Digestive biscuits, plain	1.51	
Rabbit	1.50	
Bagels	1.50	
Cherries, maraschino	1.50	
Cocoa powder	1.50	
Game meat, deer, cooked	1.50	
Strawberries, canned	1.50	
Wheat biscuits e.g. WEETABIX	1.50	
Olives, green, in brine	1.40	
Veal, mince, raw	1.40	
Radish	1.30	
Banana chips	1.30	
Salami	1.11	
Game meat, deer, raw	1.10	
Butternut squash	1.10	
Pumpkin flesh	1.10	
Ricotta cheese	1.10	
Veal, escalope, raw	1.10	
Coconut oil	1.00	
Swede	1.00	

	Vitamin K₁ µg per 100g	Vitamin K₂ µg per 100g
Taro, raw	1.00	
Worcestershire sauce	1.00	
Pate, liver	0.95	
Potatoes, old	0.94	
Fruit jam	0.90	
Instant mashed potato powder	0.90	
Spaghetti squash, raw	0.90	
Brown rice	0.82	
Ginger, ground	0.80	
Beef, rump steak, raw	0.80	
Shallots	0.80	
Spaghetti squash, baked	0.80	
Vanilla ice cream	0.80	
Plain white flour	0.76	
Beef pastrami	0.70	
Gourd	0.70	
Peanut oil (Groundnut)	0.70	
Pineapple, canned	0.70	
Plantain, raw	0.70	
Sour cream, reduced fat	0.70	
Soymilk	0.69	
Lime juice	0.60	
Caviar	0.60	
Lime, flesh	0.60	
Milk, whole	0.60	
Goat's milk	0.53	
Mango	0.52	
Salmon, farmed	0.50	0
Egg noodles, dried	0.50	
Breadfruit	0.50	
Evaporated milk	0.50	
White bread	0.42	
Onions	0.40	

	Vitamin K$_1$ µg per 100g	Vitamin K$_2$ µg per 100g
Duck eggs	0.40	
Goose eggs	0.40	
Salmon, wild	0.40	
Sweetcorn, frozen, boiled	0.40	
White wine	0.40	
Sweetcorn kernels, fresh, boiled	0.37	
Condensed milk	0.36	
Pork fat	0.35	
Dry roasted peanuts	0.31	
Cod liver oil	0.30	
Cornflour	0.30	
Peanut butter, smooth	0.30	
Quail eggs	0.30	
Rutabagas	0.30	
Salsify, flesh only	0.30	
Watermelon	0.30	
Lamb, loin chops, grilled	0.28	
Mushrooms	0.28	
Tea, black, infusion, average	0.27	
Tuna, canned in brine, drained	0.25	
Pasta, white, dried, uncooked	0.21	
Pineapple	0.21	
Baby sweetcorn, canned	0.20	
Beetroot, raw	0.20	
Long grain rice	0.20	
Pickled herring	0.20	
Pitta bread, white	0.20	
TABASCO sauce	0.20	
Water chestnuts, canned	0.20	
Beef, topside lean, roasted	0.19	
Pork fat, raw	0.18	
Pork, loin chops, lean + fat, cooked	0.16	
Turnip	0.15	

	Vitamin K₁ μg per 100g	Vitamin K₂ μg per 100g
Salmon, pink, in brine	0.10	0.5
Anchovy	0.10	
Cheese, cottage, plain, reduced fat	0.10	
Coconut milk	0.10	
Couscous, plain, cooked	0.10	
Crayfish	0.10	
Frog legs	0.10	
Ginger, fresh	0.10	
Haddock	0.10	
Halibut	0.10	
Herring	0.10	
Jerusalem artichoke	0.10	
Kohl rabi	0.10	
Mackerel	0.10	
Mullet, grey	0.10	
Mussels	0.10	
Octopus	0.10	
Orange juice, freshly squeezed	0.10	
Pollock	0.10	
Red snapper	0.10	
Sea Bass	0.10	
Snail	0.10	
Swordfish	0.10	
Trout	0.10	
Tuna, raw	0.10	
Whelks	0.10	
Whiting	0.10	
Prawns	0.08	
Bananas	0.06	
Coffee infusion	0.06	
Cornflakes	0.06	
Plantain, boiled	0.06	
Chicken, raw	0.05	

	Vitamin K$_1$ µg per 100g	Vitamin K$_2$ µg per 100g
Oranges	0.05	
Parsnips	0.05	
Pasta, white, dried, boiled	0.05	
Chicken, roasted	0.04	
Low fat yogurt	0.03	
Pork, loin chops, lean + fat, raw	0.03	
Skimmed milk	0.02	
Eggs, chicken	0.01	18
Bacon	0.01	
Beer, bitter	0.01	
Cod	0.01	
Grapefruit	0.01	
Lager	0.01	
Red wine	0.01	
Spirits, 40% volume	0.01	
Stout, GUINNESS	0.01	
Portabella mushrooms	0.00	0.3
Almond butter	0.00	
Almonds	0.00	
Bamboo shoots	0.00	
Caraway seeds	0.00	
Carob flour	0.00	
Celery seeds	0.00	
Cola	0.00	
Eel	0.00	
Fish sauce	0.00	
Grapefruit, canned	0.00	
Ham	0.00	
Honey	0.00	
Kumquats	0.00	
Lemon juice	0.00	
Lemon peel	0.00	
Lemon, flesh	0.00	

	Vitamin K_1 µg per 100g	Vitamin K_2 µg per 100g
Mandarin oranges	0.00	
Marmalade	0.00	
Nutmeg	0.00	
Oyster sauce	0.00	
Pork, lean, average, raw	0.00	
Quinoa	0.00	
Rice flour, white	0.00	
Rice noodles	0.00	
Sesame seeds	0.00	
Shitake mushrooms	0.00	
Sour cream, fat free	0.00	
Squid	0.00	
Star fruit	0.00	
Sugar, brown	0.00	
Sweetcorn kernels, canned	0.00	
Sweeteners, aspartame or saccharin	0.00	
Tapioca	0.00	
Turkey, meat, average	0.00	
Vanilla extract	0.00	

Table 2: **Protein – High to Low**

	Protein g per 100g
Gelatine	84.40
Dried egg whites	81.70
Spirulina, dried	57.47
High Protein Shake powder	53.57
Dried eggs, whole	48.60
Pork scratchings	47.90
Yeast extract e.g. MARMITE	40.70
Beef extract e.g. BOVRIL	40.40
Partridge, roasted	36.70
Beef, topside lean, roasted	36.20
Parmesan cheese, fresh	36.20
Pork crackling	36.20
Dried skimmed milk	36.10
Soya beans, dried	35.90
Yeast, dried	35.60
Soya flour	34.30
Lamb, leg + shoulder, lean, braised	33.69
Beef, braising steak, lean + fat, braised	32.90
Cheddar cheese, half fat	32.70
Seaweed, nori, dried	30.70
Goat's cheese, hard	30.52
Chicken, light meat, roasted	30.20
Emmental cheese	30.20
Lamb, loin chops, lean, grilled	29.20
Pigeon, roasted	29.00
Mustard powder	28.90
Melon seeds	28.50
Parmesan cheese, grated	28.42
Pork, loin chops, lean + fat, grilled	28.30
Ostrich, top loin, cooked	28.12

	Protein g per 100g
Pheasant, roasted	27.90
Beef, brisket, lean+ fat, boiled	27.80
Grouse, roasted	27.60
Gammon rashers, grilled	27.50
Goose, meat, fat + skin, roasted	27.50
Pollock, steamed	27.40
Wheatgerm	27.30
Gruyere cheese	27.20
Parma ham	27.20
Split black gram (urad dahl), skinned	27.20
Mung beans, dahl, dried	26.80
Edam cheese	26.70
Broad beans, dried	26.10
Paneer cheese	26.00
Split black gram (chilki urad dahl), with skin	26.00
Corned beef, canned	25.90
Port Salut cheese	25.50
Cheddar cheese	25.40
Salmon, smoked (hot-smoked)	25.40
Sardines, fresh, grilled	25.40
Duck, meat only, roasted	25.30
Gouda cheese	25.30
Tuna	25.20
Quail, cooked	25.10
Peanuts	25.00
Red Leicester cheese	25.00
Black gram, urad gram, whole	24.90
Mustard seeds, ground	24.90
Mint, dried	24.80
Beef, mince, extra lean, stewed	24.70
Caviar	24.60
Double Gloucester cheese	24.40
Pumpkin seeds	24.40

	Protein g per 100g
Lentils, green and brown, dried	24.30
Spinach, dried	24.30
Chicken, light meat, raw	24.00
Chorizo	24.00
Halloumi cheese	23.90
Mung beans, whole, dried	23.90
Beef, silverside, lean, raw	23.80
Fenugreek seeds	23.80
Red lentils, split, dried	23.80
Shrimps, boiled	23.80
Blue stilton	23.70
Wensleydale	23.70
Pink salmon, canned in brine, drained	23.60
Blackeye beans, whole, dried	23.50
Doner kebab meat	23.50
White Cheshire cheese	23.40
Gammon joint, boiled	23.30
Sardines, canned in olive oil, drained	23.30
Caerphilly cheese	23.20
Chervil, dried	23.20
Scallops, steamed	23.20
Beef, topside, lean, raw	23.00
Shark, raw	23.00
Swordfish, grilled	22.90
Peanut butter, smooth	22.80
Salmon, smoked (cold-smoked)	22.80
Tarragon, dried, ground	22.80
Gram flour	22.70
Veal, escalope, raw	22.70
Turkey meat, average, raw	22.60
Quail, breast, raw	22.59
Lamb, shoulder/stewing, lean + fat	22.50
Venison, raw	22.20

	Protein g per 100g
Lobster, boiled	22.10
Salmon, wild, raw	22.10
Sardines, canned in brine, drained	22.10
Split peas, dried	22.10
Beef, rump steak, lean, raw	22.00
Beef, mince, extra lean, raw	21.90
Rabbit	21.90
Beef, mince, stewed	21.80
Coriander leaves, dried	21.80
Pastrami	21.80
Pigeon peas, dahl, dried	21.80
Pork, lean, average, raw	21.80
Cod roe, hard	21.70
Jackfish, raw	21.70
Kippers, grilled	21.70
Beef, sirloin steak, lean + fat, raw	21.60
Dried peas	21.60
Goat's cheese, semisoft	21.58
Camembert	21.50
Halibut, raw	21.50
Haricot beans, whole, dried	21.40
Chick peas, raw	21.30
Pig liver, raw	21.30
Beef, fillet steak, lean, raw	21.20
Almonds	21.10
Mackerel, smoked	21.10
Ox liver, raw	21.10
Pinto beans, dried	21.10
Flying fish, raw	21.00
Almond butter	20.96
Beef, fillet steak, lean + fat, raw	20.90
Chicken, dark meat, raw	20.90
Salami	20.90

	Protein g per 100g
Beef, braising steak, lean + fat, raw	20.70
Beef, rump steak, raw	20.70
Tempeh	20.70
Poppy seeds	20.60
Cashew nuts, roasted, salted	20.50
Crab, white meat, cooked	20.50
Danish blue cheese	20.50
NESTLE Build up shake powder	20.50
Smoked cheese, processed	20.50
Beef, silverside, lean + fat, raw	20.40
Salmon, farmed, raw	20.40
Anchovy	20.35
Brie	20.30
Lambs liver	20.30
Mackerel, grilled	20.30
Veal, mince	20.30
Duck, meat, fat and skin, roasted	20.00
Oxtail, raw	20.00
Pigeon peas, whole, dried	20.00
Sea Bass, raw	20.00
Dill, dried	19.90
Trout, raw	19.90
White Stilton	19.90
Caraway seeds	19.80
Mullet, grey, raw	19.80
Sardines, raw	19.80
Sunflower seeds	19.80
Beef, mince, raw	19.70
Duck, meat only, raw	19.70
Langoustine, boiled	19.70
Roquefort cheese	19.70
Smoked haddock, raw	19.70
Lamb, breast, lean, raw	19.60

	Protein g per 100g
Red snapper, raw	19.60
Whelks, boiled	19.50
Pork, mince, raw	19.20
Butter beans, dried	19.10
Lamb, mince, raw	19.10
Pork, belly joint, lean + fat, raw	19.10
Poussin, meat + skin, raw	19.10
John Dory, raw	19.00
Beef, fat, average	18.90
Bacon rashers, back, fat trimmed, raw	18.80
Crab, brown meat, purchased cooked	18.80
Ling, raw	18.80
Pomfret, raw	18.80
Garlic powder	18.70
Red Mullet, raw	18.70
Whiting, raw	18.70
Lamb, chump steaks, lean + fat, raw	18.60
Mozzarella, fresh	18.60
Pork, loin chops, lean + fat, raw	18.60
Squash seeds	18.55
Goat's cheese, soft	18.52
Cocoa powder	18.50
Sardines, canned in tomato sauce	18.50
Tahini paste	18.50
Beef, brisket, lean+ fat, raw	18.40
Ham, average	18.40
Calves liver, raw	18.30
Sprats, raw	18.30
Flaxseeds	18.29
Sesame seeds	18.20
Celery seeds	18.10
Conger eel, raw	18.10
Crab, canned in brine, drained	18.10

	Protein g per 100g
Dover sole, raw	18.10
Coley, raw	18.00
Hake, raw	18.00
Mackerel, raw	18.00
Swordfish, raw	18.00
Octopus, raw	17.90
Pistachio nuts	17.90
Cumin seeds	17.80
Haddock, raw	17.80
Herring, raw	17.80
Processed cheese	17.80
Natto	17.72
Cashew nuts, plain	17.70
Chicken livers, raw	17.70
Turbot, raw	17.70
Anise seeds	17.60
Catfish, raw	17.60
King prawns, raw	17.60
Lamb, shoulder, lean + fat, raw	17.60
Carp, raw	17.50
Cod, raw	17.50
Gammon joint, raw	17.50
Sea bream, raw	17.50
Rack of lamb, lean + fat, raw	17.30
Ox kidney, raw	17.20
Burger, 98-99% beef, raw	17.10
Lambs kidney	17.00
Hoki, raw	16.90
Lamb, loin joint, lean + fat, raw	16.90
Oats	16.89
Roe, herring, soft, raw	16.80
Crayfish, cooked	16.77
Egg yolk, boiled	16.70

	Protein g per 100g
Lemon sole, raw	16.70
Pickled herring	16.70
Yellow eel, raw	16.60
Chia seeds	16.54
Goose, meat, fat + skin, raw	16.50
Shrimps, frozen	16.50
Egg yolk, raw	16.40
Flounder, raw	16.40
Frog legs, raw	16.40
Plaice, raw	16.40
Pollock, raw	16.40
Goose liver, raw	16.37
King prawns, purchased cooked	16.20
COMPLAN powder	16.10
Cuttlefish, raw	16.10
Snails, raw	16.10
Dill seeds	16.00
Eggs, whole, fried without fat	16.00
Burger, 62-85% beef, raw	15.90
Fennel seeds	15.80
Parsley, dried	15.80
Dab, raw	15.70
Ox tongue, pickled	15.70
Feta cheese	15.60
Garam masala	15.60
Pigs kidney, raw	15.50
Prawns, purchased cooked	15.40
Squid, raw	15.40
Winkles, boiled	15.40
Skate, raw	15.10
Crayfish, raw	14.90
Bran, wheat	14.80
Walnuts	14.70

	Protein g per 100g
Instant coffee powder	14.60
Quark	14.60
Mustard powder	14.50
Monkfish, raw	14.48
Basil, dried	14.40
NESTLE Build up soup powder	14.40
Sausages, pork, reduced fat, raw	14.40
Brazil nuts	14.30
Duck eggs, raw	14.30
Pork fat, cooked	14.20
Eggs, whole, boiled	14.10
Hazelnuts	14.10
Paprika	14.10
Pine nuts	14.00
Quorn pieces	14.00
Soya beans, dried	14.00
Goose eggs	13.87
Quinoa	13.80
Sausages, premium, raw	13.80
Turkey eggs, raw	13.70
Chilli powder	13.50
Dried sweetcorn	13.40
Liver sausage	13.40
Cockles in vinegar, drained	13.30
Eggs, whole, poached	13.30
Lamb, fat, average, raw	13.30
Miso	13.30
Wheat flour, whole-grain	13.21
Duck, meat, fat and skin, raw	13.10
McDONALDS Big Mac	13.10
Egg white, boiled	13.00
Egg pasta, white, raw	12.90
Quail eggs, whole, raw	12.90

	Protein g per 100g
Marjoram, dried	12.70
Sausages, beef, raw	12.70
Eggs, whole, raw	12.60
Liver pate	12.60
Wholewheat pasta, dried	12.60
Bran type cereal e.g. ALL BRAN	12.40
Coriander seeds	12.40
Seaweed, wakame, dried	12.40
Wild rice, raw	12.20
Mixed herbs, dried	12.10
Mussels, raw	12.10
Cayenne pepper	12.00
Cockles, boiled	12.00
Couscous, plain, raw	12.00
Egg noodles, dried	12.00
Sausages, pork, raw	11.90
Papadums, takeaway	11.50
Saffron	11.40
Pasta, white, dried	11.30
Breadsticks	10.90
Porridge oats	10.90
Cardamom, ground	10.80
Egg white, raw	10.80
Oysters, raw	10.80
Haggis, boiled	10.70
Cottage cheese, plain, reduced fat	10.60
Egg pasta, fresh, raw	10.60
Sage, dried, ground	10.60
Semolina, raw	10.60
Wheat, bulgur, raw	10.60
Wheat biscuits e.g. WEETABIX	10.50
Black pepper	10.40
Bread rolls, wholemeal	10.40

	Protein g per 100g
White pepper	10.40
Ginkgo nuts	10.35
Chapati flour, brown	10.30
Ciabatta	10.20
Breadcrumbs, retail	10.10
Pork, fat, average, raw	10.10
Pretzels	10.04
Bagels, plain	10.00
Bread rolls, malted wheat	10.00
Chinese mushrooms, dried	10.00
Filo pastry, cooked	10.00
Bread rolls, brown	9.90
Chapati flour, white	9.70
Chicken skin, raw	9.70
Bran flakes, fortified	9.60
Shiitake mushrooms, dried	9.60
Chinese 5 spice	9.50
Curry powder	9.50
Cottage cheese, plain	9.40
Ricotta cheese	9.40
Wholemeal bread	9.40
Bacon fat, average, cooked	9.30
Bread rolls, white	9.30
Oatcakes, plain, retail	9.30
Pecan nuts	9.20
Black pudding, raw	9.10
Pitta bread, white	9.10
Plain white flour	9.10
Thyme, dried, ground	9.10
Oregano, dried, ground	9.00
Dried onions	8.80
Lentils, green and brown, dried, boiled	8.80
Crispbread, rye	8.60

	Protein g per 100g
Chick peas, dried, boiled	8.40
Evaporated milk	8.40
Jellied eel	8.40
Broad beans, canned, drained	8.30
Split peas, dried, boiled	8.30
Wholegrain mustard	8.20
SLIMFAST Shake powder	8.13
Basmati rice, white, raw	8.10
Tofu, soya bean	8.10
White chocolate	8.00
Fava beans, raw	7.92
Bread, brown or white	7.90
Broad beans, frozen, boiled	7.90
Garlic, raw	7.90
Macadamia nuts	7.90
Pearl barley, raw	7.90
Evaporated milk, light	7.80
Malt bread, fruited	7.80
Naan bread, retail	7.80
Soft tortilla, wheat	7.80
Dark chocolate, 70-85% cacao solids	7.79
Brown rice, raw	7.70
Fromage frais, virtually fat free	7.70
Bay leaf, dried	7.60
Filo pastry, uncooked	7.60
Mung beans, whole, dried, boiled	7.60
Red split lentils, dried, boiled	7.60
Condensed milk, sweetened	7.40
Ginger, ground	7.40
Rice cakes	7.40
Scotch Pie or Bridie	7.40
Milk chocolate	7.30
Ovaltine powder	7.30

	Protein g per 100g
Puff pastry, frozen, ready-to-bake	7.30
Rye flour	7.30
Chick peas, canned, drained	7.20
Couscous, plain, cooked	7.20
Tortilla chips, fried in sunflower oil	7.20
Butter beans, dried, boiled	7.10
Cornflakes	7.10
Mustard, smooth	7.10
Seaweed, kombu, dried	7.10
Tripe, dressed, raw	7.10
Red rice, raw	7.00
Sour cream, reduced fat	7.00
Cornflour	6.93
Kidney beans, red, canned, drained	6.90
Peas, marrowfat + processed, canned, drained	6.90
Shortcrust pastry, cooked	6.90
Houmous	6.80
Long grain white rice, raw	6.70
Mace, ground	6.70
Peas, fresh	6.70
Puff pastry, cooked	6.70
Turmeric, ground	6.70
Fresh pasta, boiled	6.60
Haricot beans, whole, dried, boiled	6.60
SLIMFAST High Protein Shake, ready to drink	6.59
Biscuits, semi-sweet e.g. Rich Tea	6.40
Chocolate biscuits e.g. BREAKAWAY	6.40
Drinking chocolate powder	6.40
Rice flour	6.40
Risotto rice, Arborio, raw	6.40
Thai fragrant rice, raw	6.40
Vegetable pakora, retail	6.40
Liquorice powder	6.30

	Protein g per 100g
Chocolate nut spread	6.20
Digestive biscuits	6.20
Pinto beans, refried	6.20
Dark chocolate, 60-69% cacao solids	6.12
Allspice, ground	6.10
Cloves, dried	6.00
Corn snacks e.g. WOTSITS	6.00
Rice noodles, dry	5.95
Butter beans, canned, drained	5.90
Egg noodles, dried, boiled	5.80
Mushy peas, canned, reheated	5.80
Nutmeg, ground	5.80
Tamarind leaves, fresh	5.80
Broad beans, fresh, raw	5.70
Greek style yogurt, plain	5.70
Shortcrust pastry, uncooked	5.70
Desiccated coconut	5.60
Pesto, green	5.60
Pudding rice, raw	5.60
Pasta, white, dried, boiled	5.50
Sheep's milk, raw	5.40
Full fat soft cheese	5.30
Marzipan	5.30
Peas, canned + frozen	5.30
Puff pastry, uncooked	5.30
Baking powder	5.20
Wholewheat pasta, dried, boiled	5.20
Broad beans, fresh, boiled	5.10
Fish sauce	5.06
Arrowhead, raw	5.00
Baked beans in tomato sauce	5.00
Biscuits, cream sandwich e.g. Custard Creams	5.00
Plain chocolate, 36-50% cocoa solids	5.00

	Protein g per 100g
Yogurt	5.00
Longans, dried	4.90
Rosemary, dried	4.90
Apricots, dried	4.80
Bacon, fat only, average, raw	4.80
Ginger nut biscuits	4.80
Wasabi, root, raw	4.80
Carob flour	4.62
Mascarpone cheese	4.60
Horseradish, raw	4.50
Quinoa, cooked	4.40
Taro leaves, raw	4.40
Tomato puree	4.40
Ginkgo nuts, raw	4.32
Broccoli, raw	4.30
Potato snacks e.g. PRINGLES	4.30
Alfalfa sprouts, raw	4.10
MARS bar	4.10
Cinnamon, ground	4.00
Broccoli, purple sprouting, raw	3.90
Marshmallows	3.90
Sage, fresh	3.90
Mint, fresh	3.80
Chestnuts, dried	3.70
Dill, fresh	3.70
Figs, dried	3.60
Rocket (Arugula), raw	3.60
Amaranth leaves, raw	3.50
Brussels sprouts	3.50
Chip Shop chips	3.50
Milk, average	3.50
Radish leaves, raw	3.50
Asparagus, fresh, boiled	3.40

	Protein g per 100g
Buttermilk	3.40
Kale, raw	3.40
Mangetout	3.40
Peaches, dried	3.40
Peas, sugar-snap	3.40
Sweetcorn, kernels	3.40
Tarragon, fresh	3.40
SLIMFAST Shake regular, ready to drink	3.32
Broccoli, fresh, boiled	3.30
Chives, fresh	3.30
Dates	3.30
Figs, semi dried ready-to-eat	3.30
Single cream	3.30
Sun dried tomatoes, in oil	3.30
Coconut flesh, fresh	3.20
Basil, fresh	3.10
Goat's milk	3.10
Soymilk	3.10
Spinach, frozen, boiled	3.10
Sugar snap peas, boiled	3.10
Parsley, fresh	3.00
Probiotic milk drink e.g. YAKULT	3.00
Soy sauce, light + dark	3.00
Spring greens, raw	3.00
Thyme, fresh	3.00
Watercress, raw	3.00
Asparagus, raw	2.90
Brussels sprouts, fresh, boiled	2.90
Globe artichoke, raw	2.80
Okra, raw	2.80
Prunes	2.80
Spinach, mature, raw	2.80
Creme fraiche, half fat	2.70

	Protein g per 100g
Sultanas	2.70
Bamboo shoots, raw	2.60
Cress, garden, raw	2.60
Baby sweetcorn, fresh, boiled	2.50
Cauliflower, raw	2.50
Horseradish sauce	2.50
Potatoes, old, flesh + skin	2.50
Green cabbage, raw	2.40
Kale, fresh, boiled	2.40
Currants	2.30
Creme fraiche, full fat	2.20
Spinach, fresh, boiled	2.20
COFFEEMATE whitener	2.10
Coriander leaves, fresh	2.10
Green beans, raw	2.10
Raisins	2.10

Table 3: **Vitamin K and Protein – A to Z**

		Common Serving	Vit K mcg	Protein g	Fat g	Calories kcal
Alfalfa sprouts	raw	1 cup, 33g	10.07	1.32	0.23	8
Almond butter		1 tablespoon, 16g	0.00	3.35	8.88	98
Almonds	flaked and ground	100g	0.00	21.10	55.80	612
	toasted	6 almonds, 7g	0.00	1.55	4.14	45
Amaranth leaves ❀	raw	1 cup, 28g	319.20	0.98	0.08	5
Apple	average eating apple	medium apple, 100g	5.60	0.60	0.50	51
Apple juice	unsweetened	small glass, 150g		0.15	0.00	56
Apricots	canned in juice	1 serving, 140g	3.08	0.70	0.14	48
	canned in syrup	1 serving, 140g	3.08	0.56	0.14	88
	dried	1 average, 8g		0.38	0.06	15
	raw, flesh + skin	1 average, 40g	1.32	0.36	0.04	12
Arrowroot	powder	100g		0.40	0.10	355
Asparagus	❀ fresh, boiled	5 average spears, 120g	62.18	4.08	0.96	31
	frozen, boiled	5 average spears, 120g	96.00	3.54	0.50	22
	raw	5 average spears, 120g	49.92	3.48	0.72	30
Aubergine	raw	½ medium, 150g	9.15	1.35	0.60	23
Avocado	flesh only	small avocado, 100g	21.00	1.90	19.50	190

	Common Serving	Vit K mcg	Protein g	Fat g	Calories kcal
Bacon	back, grilled	1 rasher, 25g	0.00	5.80	5.40	72
	back, raw	1 rasher, 25g	0.00	4.13	4.13	54
	streaky, grilled	2 rashers, 25g	0.00	5.95	6.73	84
	streaky, raw	2 rashers, 25g	0.00	3.95	5.90	69
Bagels	plain	1 bagel, 85g	1.28	8.50	1.53	232
Baking powder		1 teaspoon, 5g		0.26	0.00	8
Bamboo shoots	canned, drained	100g	0.00	1.50	0.20	11
	raw	100g	0.00	2.60	0.30	27
Banana chips		10 chips, 13g	0.17	0.30	4.37	67
Banana	flesh only	medium banana, 100g	0.06	1.20	0.10	81
Barley	pearl, raw	50g serving	1.10	3.95	0.85	180
Basil	dried, ground	1 teaspoon, 1g	17.15	0.14	0.04	3
	fresh	1 large sprig, 1g	4.15	0.03	0.01	0
Bay leaf	dried	1g		0.08	0.08	3
Beans	baked, canned in tomato sauce	½ tin, 208g		10.40	1.04	168
	blackeye, whole dried	100g		23.60	1.70	312
	broad (fava), raw	100g	40.90	7.92	0.73	88
	broad, canned, drained	½ tin, 95g		7.89	0.67	83
	broad, dried	100g		26.10	2.10	245

	Common Serving	Vit K mcg	Protein g	Fat g	Calories kcal
Beans					
broad, fresh, raw	1 serving, 80g		4.56	0.80	47
broad, frozen, boiled	1 serving, 80g	9.12	6.32	0.48	65
butter, canned, drained	½ tin drained, 120g		7.08	0.60	92
butter, dried, boiled	2 tablespoons, 120g		8.52	0.72	124
butter, dried, raw	100g		19.10	1.70	290
dried, raw	100g		21.10	1.60	327
green, frozen, boiled	medium portion, 90g	7.02	1.53	0.09	23
green, raw	medium portion, 90g	35.10	1.89	0.36	22
haricot, dried, boiled	1 tablespoon, 30g		1.98	0.15	29
haricot, dried, raw	100g		21.40	1.60	286
pinto, canned, drained	100g		6.99	0.90	114
red kidney, canned, drained	½ tin drained, 120g	4.92	8.28	0.72	110
red kidney, canned, drained	400g tin drained, 240g	9.84	16.56	1.44	221
refried	100g		6.20	1.10	107
runner, fresh, boiled	medium serving, 90g	23.40	1.08	0.45	16
runner, raw	100g	26.00	1.60	0.40	22
soya, dried, raw	100g		0.00	0.00	0
Beansprouts					
mung, raw	100g	0.01	2.90	0.50	31
Beef					
braising steak, lean+fat, braised	100g	2.50	32.90	12.70	246

	Common Serving	Vit K mcg	Protein g	Fat g	Calories kcal
braising steak, lean + fat, raw	100g		20.70	8.60	160
brisket, lean+ fat, boiled	100g	1.90	27.80	17.40	268
brisket, lean+ fat, raw	100g		18.40	16.00	218
dripping	1 tablespoon, 13g	3.19	0.00	12.87	116
fillet steak, lean, raw	8oz steak, 227g		48.12	13.85	318
liver, raw	100g	3.10	21.10	7.80	155
mince, extra lean, raw	100g		21.90	4.20	130
mince, extra lean, stewed	100g		24.70	4.20	137
mince, raw	100g	2.90	19.70	16.20	225
mince, stewed	100g	7.18	21.80	13.50	209
rump steak, lean + fat, raw	8oz steak, 227g	1.82	46.99	22.93	395
silverside, 18% fat, raw	100g		20.40	14.80	215
silverside, lean, raw	100g		23.80	4.30	134
sirloin steak, lean + fat, raw	8oz steak, 227g	4.31	49.03	28.83	456
topside, lean, raw	100g		23.00	2.70	116
topside, lean, well done	medium portion, 90g	0.17	32.58	5.67	182
topside, 15% fat, raw	100g		20.40	12.90	198
Beef extract e.g. Bovril	1 level teaspoon, 9g		3.64	0.05	16
Beer average bitter (<4% ABV)	1 pint	0.06	1.70	0.00	170

		Common Serving	Vit K mcg	Protein g	Fat g	Calories kcal
Beet greens	❀ fresh, boiled	1 cup, 144g	696.96	3.70	0.29	39
	raw	1 cup, 38g	152.00	0.84	0.05	8
Beetroot	pickled, drained	1 small, 35g		0.42	0.07	10
	raw	100g	0.20	1.70	0.10	36
Bhaji	spinach + potato (homemade)	100g	284.45	3.60	14.10	192
Bicarbonate of soda		1 teaspoon		0.00	0.00	0
Biscuits	chocolate coat e.g. Breakaway	1 biscuit, 19g	0.66	1.22	5.17	96
	digestive	1 biscuit, 14.8g	0.22	0.92	3.15	69
	ginger nuts	1 biscuit, 10g	0.16	0.48	1.57	44
	sandwich e.g. Custard Cream	1 biscuit, 12.6g	0.48	0.63	2.94	60
	semi sweet e.g. Rich Tea	1 biscuit, 8.3g	0.14	0.53	1.25	37
Black gram	average, dried	100g		26.00	1.40	287
Black pepper	ground	1 teaspoon, 2g	3.27	0.21	0.07	5
Black pudding	raw	average slice, 35g		3.19	7.21	97
Blackberries	raw	small portion, 50g	9.90	0.45	0.10	13
Blackcurrants	raw	small portion, 25g		0.23	0.00	7
Blueberries	raw	small portion, 50g	9.65	0.45	0.10	20
Bran	wheat	1 tablespoon, 7g	0.73	1.04	0.39	13
Brandy	🍷	single measure, 25ml	0.04	0.00	0.00	56

	Common Serving	Vit K mcg	Protein g	Fat g	Calories kcal
Bread					
brown	1 slice, 36g		2.84	0.72	75
brown roll	1 medium, 65g		6.44	2.08	153
ciabatta	1 roll, 90g		9.18	3.51	244
malted wheat roll	1 medium, 65g		6.50	2.73	155
white	1 slice, 36g	0.15	2.84	0.58	79
white roll	1 medium, 65g		6.05	1.69	165
wholemeal	1 slice, 36g	0.72	3.38	0.90	78
wholemeal roll	1 medium, 65g		6.76	2.15	159
Breadcrumbs					
retail	10g		1.01	0.21	35
Breadfruit					
raw	1 small (edible part), 100g	0.50	1.30	0.30	95
Breadsticks					
plain	1 breadstick, 5g		0.55	0.41	19
Broccoli					
✿ fresh, boiled	1 serving, 80g	108.00	2.64	0.40	22
frozen, boiled	1 serving, 80g	70.48	2.64	0.72	25
raw	100g	185.00	4.30	0.60	34
purple sprouting, boiled	1 serving, 80g		1.68	0.48	15
purple sprouting, raw	100g		3.90	1.10	35
Brown sauce					
1 serving, 10g		0.12	0.01	10	
Brussels sprouts ✿ fresh, boiled	6 sprouts, 60g	76.20	1.74	0.78	21
fresh, raw	100g	153.00	3.50	1.40	42

	Common Serving	Vit K mcg	Protein g	Fat g	Calories kcal
Brussels sprouts frozen, boiled	6 sprouts, 60g	71.70	2.10	0.78	21
Butter	average serving, 10g	0.74	0.06	8.22	74
Cabbage green, fresh, boiled	1 serving, 90g	180.90	1.35	0.18	15
green, raw	100g	242.00	2.40	0.20	27
red, fresh, boiled	1 serving, 90g	42.84	0.72	0.27	14
red, raw	100g	38.20	1.10	0.30	21
white, fresh, boiled	1 serving, 90g	37.09	0.72	0.09	14
white, raw	100g	60.00	1.20	0.10	24
Caraway seeds dried	1 teaspoon, 1g	0.00	0.20	0.15	5
Carp raw	100g		17.50	4.70	112
Carrot juice	average serving, 160g				
Carrots frozen	100g	17.60	0.80	0.16	38
frozen, boiled	1 serving, 80g	10.88	0.78	0.46	36
old, fresh, boiled	1 serving, 80g	4.40	0.32	0.24	18
old, raw	100g	5.50	0.40	0.40	23
young, fresh, boiled	1 serving, 80g	7.36	0.50	0.40	34
young, raw	100g	9.20	0.48	0.32	18
Cashew nuts plain	10 nuts, 10g	3.41	0.70	0.50	30
roasted, salted	10 nuts, 10g	3.47	1.77	4.82	57
			2.05	5.09	61

	Common Serving	Vit K mcg	Protein g	Fat g	Calories kcal
Cassava	raw	100g	1.90	0.60	0.20	142
Catfish	raw	100g		17.60	2.80	96
Cauliflower	fresh, boiled	1 serving, 90g	25.65	1.71	0.81	26
	raw	100g	31.00	2.50	0.40	30
Cayenne pepper	ground	1 teaspoon, 1g	0.80	0.12	0.17	3
Celeriac 🌿	raw	100g	41.00	1.20	0.40	18
Celery	raw	1 stick, 30g	1.47	0.15	0.06	2
Cereal	bran flakes	1 serving, 30g		2.88	0.66	100
	bran sticks e.g. All-Bran	1 serving, 30g		3.72	1.02	80
	cornflakes, fortified	1 serving, 30g	0.02	2.13	0.24	113
	wheat biscuit e.g. Weetabix	2 biscuits, 37.5g	0.56	3.94	0.71	125
Chard, swiss 🌿	fresh, boiled	1 serving, 100g	327.30	1.90	0.10	20
	raw	100g	830.00	1.80	0.20	19
Cheese	**K2** blue	average portion, 40g	0.96	8.56	11.50	141
	Brie, rind removed	average portion, 40g	0.96	8.12	11.64	137
	Caerphilly	average portion, 40g		9.28	12.52	150
	Camembert	average portion, 40g	0.80	8.60	9.08	116
	Cheddar	average portion, 40g	1.88	10.16	13.96	166
	Cheddar, 30% less fat	average portion, 40g	0.60	11.16	8.84	126

Cheese		Common Serving	Vit K mcg	Protein g	Fat g	Calories kcal
K2	Cheddar, half fat	average portion, 40g		13.08	6.32	109
	cottage, plain	average portion, 40g		3.76	2.40	41
	cottage, plain, reduced fat	average portion, 40g	0.04	4.24	0.60	27
	Danish blue	average portion, 40g	1.64	8.20	11.56	137
	Derby	average portion, 40g		9.68	13.56	161
	Double Gloucester	average portion, 40g		9.76	14.00	165
	Edam	average portion, 40g	0.92	10.68	10.40	136
	Emmental	average portion, 40g		12.08	12.36	160
	Feta	average portion, 40g	0.72	6.24	8.08	100
	Fontina	average portion, 40g	1.04	10.24	12.46	156
	full fat soft	average portion, 40g	1.88	2.12	9.76	101
	goats, hard type	average portion, 40g	1.20	12.21	14.24	181
	goats, semisoft	average portion, 40g	1.00	8.63	11.94	146
	goats, soft	average portion, 40g	0.72	7.41	8.43	106
	Gouda	average portion, 40g	0.92	10.12	12.24	151
	Gruyere	average portion, 40g	1.08	10.88	13.32	164
	Halloumi	average portion, 40g		9.56	9.40	125
	Lancashire	average portion, 40g		9.64	12.68	153
	Mascarpone	average portion, 40g		1.84	17.80	174

	Common Serving	Vit K mcg	Protein g	Fat g	Calories kcal
Monterey	average portion, 40g	1.00	9.79	12.11	149
Mozzarella, fresh	average portion, 40g	1.00	7.44	8.12	103
Paneer	average portion, 40g		10.40	9.80	131
Parmesan, fresh	average portion, 40g		14.48	11.88	166
Parmesan, grated	1 tablespoon, 5g	0.09	1.42	1.39	21
Port Salut	average portion, 40g	0.96	10.20	10.28	133
processed, plain	average portion, 40g	0.64	7.12	9.20	119
processed, smoked	average portion, 40g		8.20	9.80	121
Provolone	average portion, 40g	0.88	10.23	10.65	140
Quark	average portion, 40g		5.84	0.00	30
Red Leicester	average portion, 40g		10.00	13.44	161
Red Windsor	average portion, 40g		9.76	13.48	160
Ricotta	average portion, 40g	0.44	3.76	4.40	58
Romano	average portion, 40g	0.88	12.72	10.78	155
Roquefort	average portion, 40g		7.88	13.16	150
Sage Derby	average portion, 40g		9.68	13.56	161
Stilton, blue	average portion, 40g		9.48	14.00	164
Stilton, white	average portion, 40g		7.96	12.52	145
Swiss	average portion, 40g	1.00	10.77	11.12	152

		Common Serving	Vit K mcg	Protein g	Fat g	Calories kcal
Cheese	K2 Wensleydale	average portion, 40g		9.48	12.72	152
	White Cheshire	average portion, 40g		9.36	12.72	152
Cherries	glace	1 serving, 25g		0.10	0.00	74
	raw, flesh + skin	4 cherries, 16g	0.34	0.14	0.02	8
Chestnuts	kernel only, raw	5 nuts, 50g		1.00	1.35	85
Chia seeds	dried	1 teaspoon, 4g		0.66	1.23	19
Chick peas	canned, drained	½ tin drained, 120g		8.64	3.48	138
	dried, boiled	1 tablespoon, 30g	0.67	2.52	0.63	36
	raw	100g	8.92	21.30	5.40	320
Chicken	dark meat, raw	100g	0.05	20.90	2.80	109
	giblets, raw	100g		18.14	5.04	127
	light meat, raw	100g	0.05	24.00	1.10	106
	light meat, roasted	100g	0.04	30.20	3.60	153
	skin, raw	100g		9.70	48.30	474
Chilli pepper	green, raw	1 medium, 9g	1.29	0.18	0.02	4
	red, raw	1 medium, 9g	1.26	0.17	0.04	4
Chilli powder		1 teaspoon, 3g	3.17	0.41	0.43	8
Chinese 5 spice	dried	1 teaspoon, 1g		0.10	0.09	2
Chives	fresh	1 tablespoon chopped, 3g	6.38	0.10	0.02	1

		Vit K mcg	Protein g	Fat g	Calories kcal
Chocolate	dark, 45-59% cacao solids	1.62	0.98	6.26	109
	dark, 60-69% cacao solids	1.44	1.22	7.66	116
	dark, 70-85% cacao solids	1.46	1.56	8.53	120
	milk		1.46	6.22	104
	plain	0.46	1.00	5.60	102
	white		1.60	6.18	106
Chocolate nut spread		0.29	0.93	4.95	82
Chorizo		0.48	7.20	9.66	119
Chutney	mango, sweet		0.14	0.02	38
Cider	dry		0.00	0.00	204
	sweet		0.00	0.00	239
Cinnamon	ground	0.94	0.12	0.04	7
Clementines	raw		0.51	0.09	28
Cocoa butter		3.46	0.00	13.93	125
Cocoa powder		0.06	0.74	0.87	12
Coconut	desiccated		5.60	62.00	604
	flesh only, fresh		3.20	36.00	351
Coconut milk	raw, fresh from coconut	0.10	0.30	0.30	22
	retail		1.10	16.90	169

Common Serving column: 1 serving, 20g; 1 serving, 20g; 1 serving, 20g; 1 serving, 20g; 1 serving, 20g; 1 serving, 20g; 1 serving, 15g; 1 small serving, 30g; 1 tablespoon, 20g; 1 pint; 1 pint; 1 teaspoon, 3g; 1 medium, 60g; 1 tablespoon, 14g; 1 teaspoon, 4g; 100g; 100g; 100ml; 100ml

		Common Serving	Vit K mcg	Protein g	Fat g	Calories kcal
Cod	raw	100g	0.01	17.50	0.60	75
Coffee	average black infusion	100ml	0.06	0.20	0.01	2
	instant, powder	1 teaspoon, 2g	0.09	0.29	0.00	2
Coffee whitener	powder	1 serving, 6g	0.36	0.13	2.07	32
Cola	average	1 can, 330ml	0.00	0.00	0.00	135
	diet	1 can, 330ml	0.00	0.00	0.00	3
Coley	raw	100g		18.00	1.10	82
Collard greens 🌿	fresh, boiled	1 serving, 130g	528.58	3.52	0.94	43
Cooking fat	solid, vegetable e.g. Trex	10g	1.38	0.00	10.00	90
Coriander	leaves, dried	1 teaspoon, 1g	13.60	0.22	0.05	3
	leaves, fresh 🌿	handful, 10g	31.00	0.21	0.05	2
	seeds	1 teaspoon, 2g		0.25	0.36	6
Corn snacks F	e.g. Wotsits	1 packet, 17g	2.64	1.02	5.17	89
Corned beef	canned	medium portion, 70g	1.40	18.13	7.63	144
Cornflour		heaped tablespoon, 30g		0.18	0.21	106
Cos lettuce 🌿	raw	1 serving, 50g	51.25	0.62	0.15	9
Courgette	raw	1 small, 100g	3.30	1.80	0.40	18
Couscous	plain, cooked	small serving, 100g	0.10	7.20	1.00	178
	plain, raw	small serving, 50g		6.00	1.05	182

	Common Serving	Vit K mcg	Protein g	Fat g	Calories kcal
Crab	brown meat, cooked	100g		18.80	7.80	145
	in brine, canned, drained	100g		18.10	0.50	77
	white meat, cooked	100g		20.50	0.30	85
Cranberries	dried, sweetened	100g	3.80	0.07	1.37	308
Cranberry juice		100ml		0.01	0.00	45
Crayfish	cooked	100g	0.10	16.77	1.20	82
	raw	100g	0.10	14.90	0.80	67
Cream	clotted, fresh	1 tablespoon, 15g		0.24	9.53	88
	double, fresh	1 tablespoon, 15g	0.96	0.24	8.06	74
	single, fresh	1 tablespoon, 15g		0.50	2.87	29
	sour, full fat	1 tablespoon, 15g	0.27	0.31	2.78	29
	sour, reduced fat	1 tablespoon, 15g	0.11	1.05	1.22	17
Cream of tartar		1 teaspoon, 5g		0.00	0.00	12
Crème fraiche	full fat	1 rounded tablespoon, 30g		0.66	12.00	113
	half fat	1 rounded tablespoon, 30g		0.81	4.50	49
Cress	garden, raw	1 tablespoon, 5g	27.10	0.13	0.04	2
	mustard and cress, raw	1 tablespoon, 5g	4.40	0.08	0.03	1
	water, raw	handful, 20g	63.00	0.60	0.20	4
Cucumber	raw	1 inch piece, 50g	10.45	0.50	0.30	7

		Common Serving	Vit K mcg	Protein g	Fat g	Calories kcal
Cumin	ground	1 teaspoon, 2g	0.11	0.36	0.45	8
	seeds	1 teaspoon, 2g	0.11	0.36	0.45	8
Curly kale	boiled	average portion, 80g	653.60	1.92	0.88	19
	raw	handful, 20g	124.60	0.68	0.32	7
Currants		1 heaped tablespoon, 25g		0.58	0.10	67
Curry powder		1 teaspoon, 1g	1.00	0.10	0.11	2
Cuttlefish	raw	100g		16.10	0.70	71
Dab	raw	100g		15.70	1.20	74
Damsons	raw, flesh + skin	100g		0.50	0.01	38
Dandelion greens	fresh, boiled	1 serving, 100g	551.40	2.00	0.60	33
	raw	large handful, 50g	389.20	1.35	0.35	23
Dates	deglet noor	1 serving, 30g	0.81	0.74	0.12	85
	dried, flesh + skin	6 dates, 42g		1.39	0.08	113
	medjool, flesh + skin	1 date, 22g	0.59	0.40	0.03	61
	raw, flesh + skin	1 date, 25g	1.40	0.38	0.03	31
Dill	dried	1 teaspoon, 1g		0.20	0.04	3
	fresh	1 sprig, 1g		0.04	0.01	0
Doner kebab meat	takeaway	small serving, 85g		19.98	26.69	320
Dover sole	raw	100g		18.10	1.80	89

	Common Serving	Vit K mcg	Protein g	Fat g	Calories kcal
Drinking chocolate powder only,	1 serving, 18g		1.15	1.04	68
Dripping beef	10g	2.45	0.00	9.90	89
Duck fat and skin, raw	100g		13.10	37.30	388
fat and skin, roasted	100g		20.00	38.10	423
meat only, raw	100g	2.80	19.70	6.50	137
meat only, roasted	100g	3.80	25.30	10.40	195
Eel conger, flesh, raw	100g	0.00	18.10	4.60	114
jellied	100g		8.40	7.10	98
yellow, raw	100g	0.00	16.60	11.30	168
Egg (Chicken) K2 white, boiled	medium 35g		4.55	0.00	18
white, dried	100g		81.70	0.01	327
white, raw	medium, 35g		3.78	0.00	15
whole, boiled	medium, 50g	0.01	7.05	4.80	72
whole, dried	100g	0.01	48.60	34.70	507
whole, fried without fat	medium, 45g		7.20	5.13	75
whole, poached	medium, 45g	0.00	5.99	4.77	67
whole, raw	medium, 50g	0.01	6.30	4.50	66
whole, scrambled without milk	medium, 45g		6.57	4.68	68
yolk, boiled	medium, 15g	0.00	2.51	4.89	54

		Common Serving	Vit K mcg	Protein g	Fat g	Calories kcal
Egg (Chicken)	K2 yolk, raw	medium, 15g	0.00	2.46	4.70	52
Egg (Duck)	whole, raw	medium, 70g	0.28	10.01	8.26	114
Egg (Goose)	whole, raw	medium, 144g	0.58	19.97	19.11	266
Egg (Quail)	whole, raw	medium, 9g	0.03	1.16	1.00	14
Egg (Turkey)	whole, raw	medium, 79g		10.82	9.64	130
Eggplant (Aubergine)	raw	½ medium, 150g	9.15	1.35	0.60	23
Elderberries	raw	100g		0.70	0.50	35
Endive	leaves, raw	1 serving, 50g	115.50	0.90	0.10	7
	bulb, raw	100g	62.80	1.24	0.20	31
Fennel	fresh, boiled	100g	4.90	0.90	0.20	11
	seeds	1 teaspoon, 1g		0.16	0.15	4
Fenugreek	seeds,	1 teaspoon, 1g		0.24	0.07	3
Figs	green raw	1 average, 55g		0.72	0.17	24
	semi dried ready-to-eat	small serving, 30g		0.99	0.45	63
	whole fruit, dried	1 fig, 9g	1.40	0.32	0.14	20
Fish sauce	ready-to-serve	1 tablespoon, 18g	0.00	0.91	0.00	6
Flaxseed	seeds	1 teaspoon, 1g	0.04	0.18	0.42	5
Flounder	raw	100g		16.40	1.80	82
Flour	cornflour	1 level tablespoon, 20g		0.12	0.14	71

	Common Serving	Vit K mcg	Protein g	Fat g	Calories kcal
gram	1 level tablespoon, 20g	1.78	4.54	1.08	71
plain	1 level tablespoon, 20g	0.15	1.82	0.28	70
rice	1 level tablespoon, 20g		1.28	0.16	73
rye	1 level tablespoon, 20g	1.18	1.46	0.32	64
soya	1 level tablespoon, 20g	5.06	6.86	4.48	82
Flying fish raw	100g		21.00	0.30	86
Frog legs raw	100g	0.10	16.40	0.30	73
Fromage frais virtually fat free	100g		7.70	0.10	49
Gammon joint boiled	100g		23.30	12.30	204
raw	100g		17.50	7.50	138
Garam masala ground	1 teaspoon, 2g		0.31	0.30	8
Garlic powder	1 teaspoon, 1g		0.19	0.01	2
raw	medium clove, 3g	0.05	0.24	0.02	3
Gelatine powder	1 sachet, 9g		7.60	0.00	30
Gherkins pickled, drained	medium, 25g		0.23	0.03	4
raw	medium, 25g		0.25	0.03	3
Gin	single measure, 25ml	0.04	0.00	0.00	52
Ginger fresh root	1 inch piece, 14g	0.01	0.25	0.11	6
ground	1 teaspoon, 2g	0.02	0.15	0.07	6

	Common Serving	Vit K mcg	Protein g	Fat g	Calories kcal
Goat	raw		20.60	2.31	109
Goose	meat, fat + skin, raw		16.50	32.80	361
	meat, fat + skin, roasted		27.50	21.20	301
Goose liver	raw	5.10	16.37	4.28	133
Gooseberries	cooking, raw		1.10	0.40	19
	dessert, raw		0.70	0.30	40
Gourd	raw	0.70	1.20	0.20	20
Grapefruit	canned in juice	0.00	0.60	0.01	30
	raw ½ grapefruit, 80g	0.01	0.64	0.08	24
Grapefruit juice	unsweetened 100ml		0.40	0.10	33
Grapes	green small bunch, 100g		0.70	0.20	62
	red small bunch, 100g		0.60	0.10	67
	red + green average small bunch, 100g	14.60	0.70	0.20	65
Green tea	infusion 100ml		0.10	0.00	1
Greengages	raw 1 medium, 50g		0.40	0.05	21
Grenadillas	flesh and seeds 100g		2.80	0.30	42
Grouse	meat only, roasted 100g		27.60	2.00	128
Guava	raw 100g	2.60	0.80	0.50	26
Haddock	raw 100g	0.10	17.80	0.40	75

	Common Serving	Vit K mcg	Protein g	Fat g	Calories kcal
smoked, raw	100g	0.10	19.70	0.50	83
Haggis boiled	100g		10.70	21.70	310
Hake raw	100g		18.00	2.20	92
Halibut raw	100g	0.10	21.50	1.90	103
Ham average	100g	0.00	18.40	3.30	107
gammon joint, boiled	100g		23.30	12.30	204
gammon joint, raw	100g		17.50	7.50	138
gammon rashers, grilled	100g		27.50	9.90	199
Herring pickled	1 roll mop, 90g	0.18	15.03	9.99	188
raw	100g	0.10	17.80	13.20	190
High Protein Shake powder 🥤	1 scoop, 25g	31.25	13.39	2.68	98
Hoki raw	100g		16.90	1.90	85
Honey	1 teaspoon, 9g	0.00	0.04	0.00	26
Horseradish raw	100g		4.50	0.30	62
Horseradish sauce	1 serving, 15g		0.38	1.26	23
Houmous	100g	3.00	6.80	26.70	307
Ice cream vanilla, non dairy	100g	0.80	2.60	7.70	192
Jackfish raw	100g		21.70	2.40	108
Jackfruit raw	100g		1.30	0.30	88

	Common Serving	Vit K mcg	Protein g	Fat g	Calories kcal
Jalapeno peppers raw	1 average, 14g	2.59	0.13	0.05	4
Jam fruit	1 serving, 15g	0.14	0.09	0.00	39
Jerusalem artichokes raw	100g	0.10	2.00	0.01	73
John Dory raw	100g		19.00	1.40	89
Kale fresh, boiled	average portion, 80g	653.60	1.92	0.88	19
frozen, boiled	average portion, 80g	705.60	2.27	0.39	24
raw	handful, 20g	124.60	0.68	0.32	7
Kelp raw	100g	66.00	1.68	0.56	43
Kidney lamb, raw	100g		17.00	2.60	91
ox, raw	100g		17.20	2.10	88
pig, raw	100g		15.50	2.70	86
Kidney Beans red, canned, drained	400g tin drained, 240g	9.84	16.56	1.44	221
Kippers flesh only, grilled	100g		21.70	17.60	245
Kiwi fruit raw, flesh + seeds	1 medium, 60g	24.18	0.66	0.30	29
Kohl rabi peeled, boiled	100g	0.10	1.20	0.20	18
peeled, raw	100g	0.10	1.60	0.20	23
Kumquats raw	1 medium, 8g	0.00	0.07	0.04	3
Lager	1 pint	0.06	1.70	0.00	136
Lamb breast, lean, raw	100g		19.60	11.20	179

	Common Serving	Vit K mcg	Protein g	Fat g	Calories kcal
chump steaks, lean + fat, raw	100g		18.60	16.40	222
fat, average, raw	100g		13.30	51.60	518
loin chops, lean, grilled	average serving, 70g	0.20	20.44	7.49	149
loin joint, lean + fat, raw	100g		16.90	26.60	307
mince, raw	100g	3.60	19.10	13.30	196
rack of, lean + fat, raw	100g		17.30	23.80	283
shoulder, lean + fat, raw	100g		17.60	18.30	235
shoulder, lean + fat, roasted	average serving, 90g	4.14	20.26	17.97	248
stewing, lean + fat, raw	100g		22.50	12.60	203
stewing, lean, braised	100g	4.40	33.69	8.80	223
Langoustine boiled	100g		19.70	0.80	86
Lard	10g		0.00	9.90	89
Leeks fresh, boiled	average portion, 75g	7.13	0.90	0.53	16
raw	1 medium leek, 90g	9.09	1.44	0.45	20
Lemon juice, bottled	1 teaspoon, 5ml	0.00	0.02	0.01	1
juice, fresh	1 teaspoon, 5ml	0.00	0.02	0.00	0
peel	1 tablespoon, 7g	0.00	0.11	0.02	3
peeled, flesh only	1 serving, 25g	0.00	0.20	0.08	4
Lemon sole raw	100g		16.70	0.70	73

	Common Serving		Vit K mcg	Protein g	Fat g	Calories kcal
Lemonade				0.01	0.00	22
raw	100ml			0.09	0.02	5
Lemongrass	1 tablespoon, 5g					
Lentils						
green + brown, boiled	1 serving, 150g			13.20	1.05	158
green + brown, raw	100g		5.00	24.30	1.90	297
red split, boiled	1 serving, 150g			11.40	0.60	150
red split, raw	100g			23.80	1.30	318
Lettuce						
average, raw	medium serving, 60g	➡	77.40	0.72	0.06	7
iceberg	medium serving, 60g		14.46	0.54	0.08	8
raddiccio	medium serving, 60g	➡	153.12	0.84	0.12	8
rocket (arugula), raw	2 handfuls, 20g	➡	21.72	0.72	0.08	4
Lime						
cordial, undiluted	1 serving, 50ml			0.05	0.00	56
juice, fresh	1 teaspoon, 5ml		0.03	0.02	0.01	0
peeled, flesh only	1 serving, 25g		0.15	0.18	0.08	2
Ling						
raw	100g			18.80	0.70	82
Liver						
calf, raw	100g			18.30	3.40	104
chicken, raw	100g			17.70	2.30	92
lamb, raw	100g			20.30	6.20	137
ox, raw	100g			21.10	7.80	155
pig, raw	100g			21.30	3.10	113

	Common Serving	Vit K mcg	Protein g	Fat g	Calories kcal
Liver sausage	average slice, 12.5g		1.68	2.09	28
Lobster boiled	100g		22.10	1.60	103
Loganberries raw	100g		1.10	0.01	17
Lychees raw, flesh only	1 average, 15g		0.14	0.02	9
Mackerel raw	100g	0.10	18.00	17.90	233
smoked	100g	0.10	21.10	24.10	301
Malted fruit loaf	1 slice, 27g		2.11	0.62	80
Mangetout fresh, boiled	average serving, 60g	9.00	1.92	0.06	16
Mango raw, flesh only	100g	0.52	0.70	0.20	57
Maple syrup canadian	1 tablespoon, 15g		0.00	0.03	39
Margarine baking, hard block	10g		0.01	7.64	69
Marjoram dried	1 teaspoon, 1g	6.22	0.13	0.07	3
Marmalade	1 serving, 15g	0.00	0.02	0.00	39
Marrow fresh, boiled	average serving, 65g	1.56	0.26	0.13	6
raw	100g		0.50	0.20	12
MARS bar	1 bar, 51g	2.45	2.09	7.80	206
Marshmallows	1 sweet, 7g		0.27	0.00	23
Marzipan white and yellow, retail	100g		5.30	12.70	389
Mayonnaise F reduced fat, retail	1 tablespoon, 14g	7.52	0.14	3.93	40

		Common Serving	Vit K mcg	Protein g	Fat g	Calories kcal
Mayonnaise	F standard, retail	1 tablespoon, 14g	22.82	0.15	10.47	96
Melon	canteloupe, flesh only	100g	2.50	0.60	0.10	19
	galia, flesh only	100g		0.50	0.10	24
	honeydew, flesh only	100g	2.90	0.50	0.10	29
Milk	coconut, raw, fresh from nut	100ml	0.10	0.30	0.30	22
	coconut, retail	100ml		1.10	16.90	169
	condensed	100g	0.36	7.40	8.00	310
	dried, fortified	1 teaspoon, 3g		10.83	0.18	104
	evaporated	100g	0.50	8.40	9.40	166
	evaporated, light	100g		7.80	4.10	107
	goats	100ml	0.53	3.10	3.70	62
	semi-skimmed	100ml		3.50	1.70	46
	skimmed	100ml	0.02	3.50	0.30	34
	soy, sweetened, fortified	100ml	0.69	3.10	2.40	43
	soy, unsweetened, fortified	100ml	1.71	2.40	1.60	26
	whole	100ml	0.60	3.40	3.60	63
Mincemeat	from jar	1 tablespoon, 24g		0.14	1.03	66
Mint	dried	1 teaspoon, 1g		0.25	0.05	3
	fresh	1 tablespoon chopped, 4g		0.15	0.03	2

	Common Serving	Vit K mcg	Protein g	Fat g	Calories kcal
	sauce	medium serving, 15g		0.24	0.00	15
Miso	paste	1 tablespoon, 18g	5.27	2.39	1.12	37
Mixed herbs	dried	1 teaspoon, 1g		0.12	0.09	3
Molasses		100g		0.00	0.10	266
Monkfish	raw	100g		14.48	1.52	76
Mullet, grey	raw	100g	0.10	19.80	4.00	115
Mung beansprouts	raw	1 handful, 40g	13.20	1.22	0.07	12
Mushrooms	chanterelle, raw	100g		1.49	0.53	38
	chinese, dried	100g		10.00	1.80	284
	oyster, raw	100g		1.60	0.20	8
	portabella, raw	100g	0.00	2.11	0.35	22
	shiitake, dried	100g	0.00	9.60	1.00	296
	shiitake, raw	100g		2.24	0.49	34
	white, raw	100g	0.28	1.00	0.20	7
Mussels	raw	100g	0.10	12.10	1.80	74
Mustard	English, retail	average serving, 5g		0.36	0.41	7
	powder, retail	1 teaspoon, 1g		0.29	0.29	5
	seeds, ground	1 teaspoon, 1g	0.05	0.25	0.29	5
	wholegrain, retail	average serving, 5g		0.41	0.51	7

	Common Serving	Vit K mcg	Protein g	Fat g	Calories kcal
Mustard and cress raw	1 tablespoon, 5g	4.40	0.08	0.03	1
Mustard greens 🌱 leaves, fresh, boiled	medium portion, 90g	533.43	2.30	0.42	23
raw	100g	257.50	2.86	0.42	27
Naan bread retail	100g	3.80	7.80	7.30	285
Natto **K2**	100g	23.10	17.72	11.00	212
Nectarines raw, flesh + skin	1 medium, 90g	2.25	1.26	0.09	36
Nettles 🌱 blanched	100g	498.60	2.71	0.11	42
Noodles egg, dried, boiled	average serving, 125g		7.25	1.25	208
egg, dried, uncooked	100g	0.50	12.00	2.00	338
fine rice, dried, boiled	average serving, 100g		1.90	0.20	89
Nutmeg ground	1 teaspoon, 1g	0.00	0.06	0.36	5
Nuts brazil, kernels	3 nuts, 15g		2.15	10.23	102
cashew, plain	10 nuts, 10g	3.41	1.77	4.82	57
cashew, roasted, salted	10 nuts, 10g	3.47	2.05	5.09	61
ginko, dried	100g		10.35	2.00	348
ginko, raw	100g		4.32	1.68	182
hazelnuts, kernels	10 nuts, 10g	1.42	1.41	6.35	65
macadamia, salted	6 whole nuts, 10g		0.79	7.76	75
peanuts, dry roasted	small bag, 50g	0.16	12.85	24.90	295

	Common Serving	Vit K mcg	Protein g	Fat g	Calories kcal
peanuts, plain	small bag, 50g		12.90	23.00	282
peanuts, roasted and salted	small bag, 50g		12.35	26.50	301
pecan, kernel only	1 whole nut, 6g	0.21	0.55	4.21	41
pine, kernel only	1 serving, 25g	13.48	3.50	17.15	172
pistachio, kernel only, roasted	10 kernels, 7g	0.92	1.25	3.88	42
walnuts, kernel only	6 halves, 20g	0.54	2.94	13.70	138
Oat bran raw	average portion, 40g	1.28	6.92	2.81	98
Octopus raw	100g	0.10	17.90	1.30	83
Oils almond	1 tablespoon, 14g	0.98	0.00	14.00	124
cocoa butter	1 tablespoon, 14g	3.46	0.00	13.93	125
coconut	1 tablespoon, 14g	0.14	0.00	13.99	126
cod liver	1 tablespoon, 14g	0.04	0.00	13.99	126
corn	1 tablespoon, 14g	0.42	0.00	13.99	126
cottonseed	1 tablespoon, 14g	3.46	0.00	13.86	125
evening primrose	1 tablespoon, 14g		0.00	13.99	126
flaxseed	1 tablespoon, 14g	1.30	0.02	14.00	124
grapeseed	1 tablespoon, 14g		0.00	13.99	126
hazelnut	1 tablespoon, 14g		0.00	13.99	126
olive	1 tablespoon, 14g	8.05	0.00	13.99	126

	Common Serving	Vit K mcg	Protein g	Fat g	Calories kcal
Oils palm	1 tablespoon, 14g	1.11	0.00	13.99	126
peanut (groundnut)	1 tablespoon, 14g	0.10	0.00	13.99	126
rapeseed (canola)	1 tablespoon, 14g	15.75	0.00	13.99	126
safflower	1 tablespoon, 14g	0.48	0.00	13.99	126
sesame	1 tablespoon, 14g	1.90	0.03	13.96	126
soya	1 tablespoon, 14g	18.34	0.00	13.99	126
sunflower	1 tablespoon, 14g	0.88	0.00	13.99	126
vegetable	1 tablespoon, 14g	15.75	0.00	13.99	126
walnut	1 tablespoon, 14g	2.10	0.00	13.99	126
wheatgerm	1 tablespoon, 14g		0.00	13.99	126
Okra boiled	3 medium, 15g	6.00	0.38	0.14	4
raw	100g	31.30	2.80	1.00	31
Olives in brine, drained, flesh + skin	100g	1.40	0.90	11.00	103
Onions dried	100g	3.80	8.80	1.20	309
pickled, drained	100g		0.90	0.20	24
raw	100g	0.40	1.00	0.10	35
Orange juice freshly squeezed	100ml	0.10	0.60	0.01	33
Oranges raw, peeled	1 medium, 160g	0.08	1.28	0.32	58
Oregano dried, ground	1 teaspoon, 2g	12.43	0.18	0.09	5

		Common Serving	Vit K mcg	Protein g	Fat g	Calories kcal
	fresh	100g		1.80	0.90	66
Oxtail	raw	100g		20.00	10.10	171
Oysters	raw	1 medium, 10g		1.08	0.13	7
Pak Choi	raw	100g	45.50	1.50	0.20	13
	steamed	3 heaped tablespoons, 80g	27.20	1.20	0.08	11
Papaya	raw, flesh only	100g	2.60	0.50	0.10	36
Paprika	dried	1 teaspoon, 1g	0.80	0.14	0.13	3
Parsley	dried	1 teaspoon, 1g	13.60	0.16	0.07	2
	fresh	1 tablespoon chopped, 4g	21.92	0.12	0.05	1
Parsnips	boiled	medium serving, 65g	0.65	1.04	0.78	43
	raw	100g	0.05	1.80	1.10	64
Passion fruit	flesh + pips	1 average, 15g		0.39	0.06	5
Pasta	egg, dried, uncooked	100g		12.90	3.60	365
	egg, fresh, raw	100g		10.60	2.90	282
	plain, fresh, boiled	medium serving, 170g		11.22	2.55	270
	white, dried, boiled	medium serving, 170g		9.35	1.36	287
	white, dried, uncooked	100g	0.21	11.30	1.60	343
	white, spaghetti, boiled	100g	0.05	4.40	0.60	141
	white, spaghetti, uncooked	100g	0.21	11.30	1.60	343

	Common Serving	Vit K mcg	Protein g	Fat g	Calories kcal
Pasta					
wholewheat, dried, boiled	medium serving, 170g		8.84	1.87	228
wholewheat, dried, uncooked	100g		12.60	2.50	329
Pastry					
filo, cooked	100g		10.00	3.80	363
filo, uncooked	100g		7.60	2.90	278
flaky, cooked	100g		5.70	37.40	540
flaky, uncooked	100g		4.30	28.30	409
puff, cooked	100g		6.70	33.20	486
puff, frozen, ready-to-bake	100g	16.10	7.30	38.10	551
puff, uncooked	100g		5.30	26.20	384
shortcrust, cooked	100g		6.90	37.90	547
shortcrust, uncooked	100g		5.70	31.40	453
wholemeal, cooked	100g		8.30	30.00	487
wholemeal, uncooked	100g		7.20	25.90	421
Pate					
liver, average	100g	0.95	12.60	32.70	349
Peaches					
dried	100g		3.40	0.80	219
raw, flesh + skin	1 medium, 110g	6.38	1.10	0.11	36
Peanut butter					
smooth	1 serving, 15g	0.05	3.42	7.77	91
Pears					
raw, flesh + skin	1 average, 133g	4.79	0.40	0.13	57
Peas					
canned	medium portion, 70g	21.28	3.71	0.63	41

	Common Serving	Vit K mcg	Protein g	Fat g	Calories kcal
fresh, boiled	medium portion, 70g	27.30	4.69	1.12	55
frozen, boiled	medium portion, 70g	16.80	3.85	0.49	49
frozen, raw	100g	27.90	5.30	0.70	68
mange-tout, fresh, boiled	average serving, 60g	9.00	1.92	0.06	16
mange-tout, raw	100g		3.60	0.20	32
marrowfat, canned, drained	average serving, 65g		4.49	0.52	57
mushy, canned	average portion, 80g	18.00	4.64	0.56	65
pigeon, dried, uncooked	100g		21.80	1.90	324
processed, canned, drained	100g		6.90	0.70	99
raw	100g	39.00	6.90	1.50	83
split, dried, raw	100g	14.50	22.10	2.40	328
sugar-snap, boiled	average serving, 60g		1.86	0.18	20
sugar-snap, raw	100g		3.40	0.20	34
Pepper black	1 teaspoon, 2.4g	3.93	0.25	0.08	6
white	1 teaspoon, 2.4g		0.25	0.05	7
Peppers chilli, red, raw	1 medium, 9g	1.26	0.17	0.04	4
green, raw	1 medium, 160g	10.24	1.28	0.48	24
jalapeno, raw	1 average, 14g	2.59	0.13	0.05	4
red, raw	1 medium, 160g	2.56	1.28	0.32	34

	Common Serving	Vit K mcg	Protein g	Fat g	Calories kcal
Peppers	yellow, raw	1 medium, 160g		1.28	0.32	37
Pesto	green	1 level tablespoon, 15g		0.84	6.38	63
	red	1 level tablespoon, 15g		0.75	4.59	48
Physalis	raw	1 average, 3g		0.05	0.01	2
Pineapple	dried	100g		2.50	1.30	276
	flesh, raw	100g	0.21	0.40	0.20	41
Pitta bread	white	1 medium, 60g	0.12	5.46	0.72	165
	wholewheat	1 medium, 60g	0.84	5.88	1.56	160
Plaice	raw	100g		16.40	1.20	76
Plantain	fresh, flesh only, boiled	100g	0.06	0.80	0.20	112
	green flesh, raw	100g	0.70	1.10	0.30	117
Plums	raw, flesh + skin	1 medium, 55g	4.13	0.33	0.06	20
Polenta	cooked in water	100g		1.90	0.40	68
Pollock	raw	100g	0.10	16.40	0.70	72
Pomegranate	flesh and pips	1 medium, 155g	25.42	2.02	0.31	79
Poppy seeds		1 tablespoon, 12g		2.47	5.65	63
Pork	average lean, raw	100g	0.00	21.80	4.00	123
	belly joint, lean + fat, raw	100g		19.10	20.20	258
	crackling, cooked	100g		36.20	45.00	550

		Common Serving	Vit K mcg	Protein g	Fat g	Calories kcal
fat, cooked		100g	0.35	14.20	50.90	515
fat, raw		100g	0.18	10.10	56.40	548
loin chops, lean + fat, cooked		1 average, 90g	0.14	25.47	14.22	230
loin chops, lean + fat, raw		100g	0.03	18.60	21.70	270
mince, raw		100g		19.20	9.70	164
scratchings		small bag, 20g		9.58	9.20	121
Porridge oats						
unfortified, not made up		average serving, 30g		3.27	2.43	114
Port						
◁◫		small glass, 50ml		0.05	0.00	79
Potato						
chips, chip shop,	F	medium portion, 368g		12.88	30.91	788
chips, frozen, fried in oil	F	medium serving, 165g		6.77	22.28	450
chips, homemade	F	medium serving, 165g		5.28	11.06	325
chips, oven ready, average	F	medium serving, 165g		5.28	8.09	312
instant mash, made with water		100g	0.90	1.50	0.10	57
new, flesh + skin, boiled		medium serving, 175g		3.15	0.18	119
new, flesh only, raw		100g		1.70	0.10	68
old, flesh + skin, baked		1 medium, 180g	1.69	4.50	0.36	175
old, flesh only, baked		1 medium, 180g	1.69	3.96	0.18	139
old, flesh only, raw		100g	0.94	1.90	0.10	82
red, flesh + skin, baked		1 medium, 180g	5.04	4.14	0.27	160

		Common Serving	Vit K mcg	Protein g	Fat g	Calories kcal
Potato	red, flesh + skin, raw	100g	2.90	1.89	0.14	70
Potato snacks F	snacks, pringle-type	1 serving, 25g	2.40	1.08	7.95	130
Poussin	meat + skin, raw	100g		19.10	13.90	202
Prawns	cooked	average serving, 75g	0.06	11.55	0.68	53
	king, cooked	6 prawns, 48g		7.78	0.19	33
	king, raw	6 prawns, 48g		8.45	0.34	37
Prunes	canned in juice	100g		0.70	0.20	79
	dried, flesh + skin	5 prunes, 45g	26.78	1.26	0.23	72
	semi dried, ready-to-eat	4 prunes, 40g		1.00	0.16	56
	stewed no sugar, flesh + skin	6 prunes, 60g	15.66	0.84	0.18	49
Pumpkin	flesh, raw	100g	1.10	0.70	0.20	13
	seeds	1 tablespoon, 15g		3.66	6.84	85
Quail	cooked	100g	4.20	25.10	14.10	227
	raw	100g		22.59	2.99	123
Quinoa	cooked	average serving, 125g	0.00	5.50	2.40	150
	dried, uncooked	100g	0.00	13.80	5.00	309
Rabbit	raw	100g		21.90	5.50	137
Radish	leaves, raw	100g		3.50	0.50	33
	red, flesh + skin, raw	1 average, 8g	0.10	0.06	0.02	1

	Common Serving	Vit K mcg	Protein g	Fat g	Calories kcal
	white/mooli, raw	1 average, 8g	0.10	0.06	0.01	1
Raisins	average	1 tablespoon, 30g	1.11	0.63	0.12	82
Raspberries	raw	15 raspberries, 60g	4.68	0.84	0.18	15
Red snapper	raw	100g	0.10	19.60	1.30	90
Redcurrants	raw	100g		1.10	0.01	21
Rhubarb	stalks, raw	100g	29.30	0.90	0.10	7
Rice	basmati, brown, raw	100g		8.90	3.10	355
	basmati, white, raw	100g		8.10	0.50	351
	brown, wholegrain, raw	100g	0.82	7.70	1.50	333
	easy cook, brown, raw	100g		7.50	3.10	366
	flour, white	100g	0.00	5.95	1.42	366
	Italian Arborio risotto, raw	100g		6.40	1.00	354
	long grain, white, raw	100g	0.20	6.70	1.00	355
	noodles, dry	100g	0.00	5.95	0.56	364
	pudding, raw	100g		5.60	0.90	352
	red, raw	100g		7.00	2.90	356
	Thai fragrant, raw	100g		6.40	1.10	352
	wild, raw	100g	1.90	12.20	1.10	343
Rocket	raw	2 handfuls, 20g	21.72	0.72	0.08	4

	Common Serving	Vit K mcg	Protein g	Fat g	Calories kcal
Romaine lettuce raw	1 serving, 50g	51.25	0.62	0.15	9
Rosemary dried	1 teaspoon, 1g		0.05	0.15	3
fresh	1 large sprig, 1g		0.01	0.04	1
Rum	single measure, 25ml	0.04	0.00	0.00	56
Saffron dried	1 teaspoon, 1g		0.11	0.06	3
Sage dried, ground	1 teaspoon, 1g	17.15	0.11	0.13	3
fresh	1 large sprig, 1g		0.04	0.05	1
Salad cream average	1 tablespoon, 15g		0.23	4.01	49
reduced fat	1 tablespoon, 15g		0.15	1.59	24
Salami	4 average slices, 20g	0.22	4.18	7.84	88
Salmon farmed, raw	100g	0.50	20.40	15.00	217
in brine, canned, drained	100g	0.10	23.60	4.80	138
smoked (cold-smoked),	100g		22.80	10.10	184
smoked (hot-smoked),	100g		25.40	8.80	186
wild, raw	100g	0.40	22.10	10.10	179
Salsify flesh only, boiled	100g	0.30	1.10	0.40	23
Salt	100g		0.00	0.00	0
Sardines canned in brine, drained	100g		22.10	9.10	170
canned in oil, drained F	100g	2.60	24.62	11.45	208

	Common Serving	Vit K mcg	Protein g	Fat g	Calories kcal
in tomato sauce, canned	100g		18.50	10.80	175
raw	100g		19.80	6.10	134
Sausages beef, raw	100g		12.70	19.50	258
pork, raw	100g		11.90	25.00	309
Scallops steamed	100g	0.00	23.20	1.40	118
Sea Bass raw	100g	0.10	20.00	9.80	168
Sea bream raw	100g		17.50	2.90	96
Seaweed 🦐 kelp, raw	100g	66.00	1.68	0.56	43
kombu, dried, raw	100g		7.10	1.60	43
nori, dried, raw	100g		30.70	1.50	136
spirulina, dried, raw	100g	25.50	57.47	7.72	290
wakame, dried, raw	100g		12.40	2.40	71
Semolina raw	100g		10.60	1.60	349
Sesame seeds	1 tablespoon, 12g	0.00	2.18	6.96	72
Shallots raw	1 medium, 20g	0.16	0.30	0.04	4
Shark raw	100g		23.00	1.10	102
Sherry 🍷 dry	single measure, 50ml		0.10	0.00	58
sweet	single measure, 50ml		0.15	0.00	68
Shrimps boiled	100g		23.80	2.40	117

	Common Serving	Vit K mcg	Protein g	Fat g	Calories kcal
Shrimps	frozen		16.50	0.80	73
Skate	raw		15.10	0.40	64
Snail	raw	0.10	16.10	1.40	90
Soda water	250ml		0.00	0.00	0
Soy sauce	light + dark, 1 tablespoon, 15g		0.45	0.00	12
Soya beans	dried, raw		35.90	18.60	370
Spinach 🌿	fresh, boiled average serving, 90g	517.50	1.98	0.72	17
	frozen, boiled average serving, 90g	756.00	2.79	0.72	19
	raw 1 handful, 25g	98.50	0.70	0.20	6
Spirits, 40% volume🥃	average single measure, 25ml	0.04	0.00	0.00	56
Spirulina	dried	25.50	57.47	7.72	290
Sprats	raw		18.30	11.00	172
Spring greens 🌿	boiled average portion, 90g	803.70	1.71	0.63	18
Spring onions 🌿	bulbs and tops, raw 3 average, 30g	62.10	0.60	0.15	7
Squash	butternut, baked ¼ average, 95g	0.95	0.86	0.10	30
	butternut, raw 100g	1.10	1.10	0.10	36
	seeds, roasted 100g		18.55	19.40	446
	spaghetti, baked 100g	0.80	0.70	0.30	23
	spaghetti, raw 100g	0.90	0.60	0.60	26

		Common Serving	Vit K mcg	Protein g	Fat g	Calories kcal
	winter, baked	average portion, 95g	4.18	1.05	0.10	53
	winter, raw	100g	4.40	0.80	0.10	40
Squid	raw	100g	0.00	15.40	1.70	81
Stout	e.g. Guiness	1 pint	0.06	2.27	0.06	210
Strawberries	raw	8 average, 100g	3.00	0.60	0.50	30
Sugar	brown	1 heaped teaspoon, 6g	0.00	0.01	0.00	23
	white	1 heaped teaspoon, 6g		0.00	0.00	24
Sultanas		1 tablespoon, 30g		0.81	0.12	83
Sunflower seeds		1 tablespoon, 16g		3.17	7.60	92
Swede	boiled	medium serving, 60g	0.60	0.18	0.06	7
	raw	100g	2.00	0.70	0.30	24
Sweet potato	baked	1 medium, 114g	2.62	1.82	0.46	131
	flesh only, boiled	medium serving, 175g	3.68	1.93	0.53	147
	flesh only, raw	100g	1.80	1.20	0.30	87
Sweetcorn	baby, fresh, boiled	5 babycorns, 65g		1.63	0.26	16
	kernels, canned, drained	average portion, 85g	0.00	2.21	1.45	66
	kernels, fresh, boiled	average portion, 85g	0.31	3.06	1.62	57
	kernels, frozen, boiled	average portion, 85g	0.34	2.64	0.63	80
	kernels, raw	100g		3.40	1.80	60

	Common Serving	Vit K mcg	Protein g	Fat g	Calories kcal
Sweetcorn on the cob, fresh, boiled	100g weighed with core	0.22	2.10	1.10	39
on the cob, raw	100g weighed with core		2.00	1.10	36
Swiss chard fresh, boiled	1 serving, 100g	327.30	1.90	0.10	20
raw	100g	830.00	1.80	0.20	19
Swordfish raw	100g	0.10	18.00	4.10	109
Syrup golden	1 tablespoon, 15g		0.05	0.00	45
maple	1 tablespoon, 15g		0.00	0.03	39
Tahini paste sesame seed pulp	100g		18.50	58.90	607
Tapioca raw	100g	0.00	0.40	0.10	359
Taro leaves, raw	100g	108.60	4.40	0.90	35
raw	100g	1.00	1.40	0.20	106
Tarragon dried, ground	1 teaspoon, 1g		0.23	0.07	3
fresh	1 large sprig, 1g		0.03	0.01	0
Tea average black infusion	100ml	0.27	0.10	0.01	0
green infusion	100ml		0.10	0.00	0
Thyme dried, ground	1 teaspoon, 1g	17.15	0.09	0.07	3
fresh	1 large sprig, 1g		0.03	0.03	1
Tofu soya bean curd, steamed	100g	2.40	8.10	4.20	73
Tomato ketchup	average serving, 10g		0.16	0.01	12

	Common Serving	Vit K mcg	Protein g	Fat g	Calories kcal
Tomatoes	canned	6.00	1.10	0.10	19
	cherry, raw	4 average, 60g		0.66	0.30	13
	juice	100ml	2.30	0.80	0.01	14
	puree, double concentrate	1 tablespoon, 15g	0.51	0.66	0.03	10
	raw	average slice, 17g	1.02	0.09	0.02	2
Tongue	lamb, raw	100g		15.30	14.60	193
	ox, pickled, raw	100g		15.70	17.50	220
Tortilla	chips, fried in sunflower oil	average serving, 40g	8.36	2.88	10.96	202
	wrap, white, soft	1 large, 64g		4.99	3.65	182
Treacle		100g		1.20	0.00	257
Tripe	dressed, raw	100g		7.10	0.50	33
Trout	brown, raw	100g	0.10	19.40	3.80	112
	rainbow, raw	100g	0.10	19.90	5.30	127
Tuna	canned in brine	100g	0.25	24.90	1.00	109
	fresh, raw	100g	0.10	25.20	0.70	107
	in sunflower oil, can, drained F	100g		25.40	6.40	159
Turbot	raw	100g		17.70	2.70	95
Turkey	average, raw	100g	0.00	22.60	1.60	105
Turmeric	ground	1 teaspoon, 3g	0.40	0.20	0.21	9

		Common Serving	Vit K mcg	Protein g	Fat g	Calories kcal
Turnip	flesh only, boiled	medium serving, 60g	0.09	0.36	0.12	7
	flesh only, raw	100g	0.15	0.90	0.30	23
Veal	escalope, raw	100g	1.10	22.70	1.70	106
	mince, raw	100g	1.40	20.30	7.00	144
Venison	raw	100g	1.10	22.20	1.60	103
Vinegar	balsamic	1 tablespoon, 15g		0.07	0.03	14
	cider	1 tablespoon, 15g		0.00	0.00	3
	distilled	1 tablespoon, 15g		0.00	0.02	3
	red wine	1 tablespoon, 15g		0.01	0.02	3
Vodka		single measure, 25ml	0.04	0.00	0.00	52
Water chestnuts	raw	100g		1.40	0.20	46
Watercress	raw	handful, 20g	63.00	0.60	0.20	4
Watermelon	flesh	100g	0.30	0.50	0.30	31
Wheat, bulgur	raw	100g		10.60	2.00	352
Wheatgerm		100g		27.30	8.40	352
Whelks	boiled	1 whelk, 7g	0.01	1.37	0.08	6
Whisky		single measure, 25ml	0.04	0.00	0.00	56
Whitecurrants	raw	100g		1.30	0.01	26
Whiting	raw	100g	0.10	18.70	0.70	81

	Common Serving	Vit K mcg	Protein g	Fat g	Calories kcal
Wine red	small glass, 175ml	0.02	0.18	0.00	133
rose	small glass, 175ml		0.18	0.00	138
white	small glass, 175ml	0.70	0.18	0.00	131
Winkles boiled, meat only	100g		15.40	1.20	72
Worcestershire sauce	1 serving, 5ml	0.05	0.07	0.01	6
Yam raw, flesh only	100g	2.30	1.50	0.30	114
Yeast dried	100g		35.60	1.50	169
Yeast extract e.g. Marmite	1 serving, 4g		1.63	0.02	7
Yoghurt greek style, plain	average serving, 120g		6.84	12.24	160
low fat, fruit	average serving, 120g	0.04	5.04	1.32	94
low fat, plain	average serving, 120g	0.04	5.76	1.20	68
virtually fat free/diet, plain	average serving, 120g		6.48	0.24	65
whole milk, plain	average serving, 120g		6.84	3.60	95

Key to Tables

0.0   Where the content has been entered as 0.00, analysis has been carried out and no significant quantity of the nutrient has been found.

blank Where values are missing from the table, no data is available. The nutrient may, or may not, be present in significant quantities but there is currently no analysis for this.

High in Vitamin K – be aware of the amount you consume. Remember, an increased amount of Vitamin K can lower your INR making Warfarin less effective and potentially increasing the risk of blood clots.

Has been linked with an increased risk of bleeding in Warfarin users – consume in moderation.

F   Be aware of the type of fat/oil used in preparation of a foodstuff. Where Vitamin K rich fats or oils have been used, the Vitamin K content of the foodstuff could be significantly increased – see Oils for comparisons

K2   Vitamin K_2 may be present in significant quantities

Please remember:

1. The availability of Vitamin K data is limited. There may be foods not recorded in these tables that contain significant amounts of Vitamin K.

2. For branded products, the most reliable nutrient and ingredient data will be on the packaging, or available from the manufacturer.

3. Watch out for hidden oils that may be high in Vitamin K e.g. in dressings, processed foods, fast foods (burgers etc.).

The majority of the values in these tables have been sourced from McCance and Widdowson's The Composition of Foods Integrated Dataset 2015 published by Public Health England. Where no UK data exists, the USDA Nutrient Database for Standard Reference Release 27 has been used.

For a downloadable food diary to help you track your Vitamin K and protein intake go to www.eatonwarfarin.com.

CHAPTER 6

The Diet I Follow

With so many options to choose from, deciding on the most suitable diet for your needs is never easy. However, when you are a Warfarin user, finding **the right diet** is a whole lot harder.

There are countless diets aimed at weight loss but, to date, I have not come across any diet which takes into consideration whether the eating regime being suggested is suitable for someone taking warfarin.

The foods specified in the majority of diets are included for one, or more, of the following reasons,

- they have a high water content

- they are high in fibre

- they add volume to meals without adding empty calories

- they slow down digestion

- they make us feel fuller for longer

- they contain nutrients which are beneficial to health

None of these are bad things. Quite the contrary, they all help to contribute towards healthy weight loss. The problem is that so many of the foods in these categories need to be **approached with**

caution by someone on Warfarin and certainly <u>not eaten in the large quantities</u> very often recommended in these diets.

For example,

Broccoli has high water and dietary fibre content and provides many important nutrients – but it is also **<u>high</u> in Vitamin K**! Similarly, **spinach** *curbs cravings*, due to its' green leaf membranes which slow down digestion, and it also has fantastic properties for health - but it has a <u>very high</u> Vitamin K content.

Protein is recommended in large quantities in some diets, such as the Atkins diet, because it helps you feel fuller for longer, curbs cravings and fuels fat burning - but **too much protein can bring about a decrease in INR**.

I learned most of this the hard way, having had many setbacks on the road to 'weight loss'. The good news is that I have managed to find a diet for myself that has allowed me to <u>lose weight while taking Warfarin</u>. Along the way I have discovered many alternative foods that I can substitute which provide **the same health benefits as the 'green**

superfoods', <u>without</u> affecting my INR.

Having recovered from my last weight loss attempt, when my INR dropped drastically as a result of eating **large amounts of protein**, I decided to take stock of exactly what it was I wanted to achieve.

My aims were as follows,

To lose weight and maintain that weight loss

To keep my INR stable

To eat 'clean' i.e. avoid processed foods and eat as much fresh food as possible

To eliminate gluten from my diet to support my immune health

Knowing that consistency was going to be crucial to keeping my INR stable, the first thing I did was to set *<u>suitable targets</u>* for the amount of **Vitamin K** and **Protein** I wanted to be consuming daily.

For Vitamin K the UK recommended daily allowance for the average woman is 75mcg (or 0.000075g). These <u>RDAs are the minimum</u> that our bodies should be getting and, being mindful of the **importance of**

Vitamin K to health, I decided to set *my* **daily target at 150mcg**.

For my Protein target, not wanting to repeat my earlier mistakes, I decided to stay close to the UK recommended daily intake for the average woman of 45g and set *my* **daily target at 50g.**

I discussed these targets with my doctor who was happy that, as long as I <u>maintained consistency</u> and my **INR was closely monitored** to start with, there should be no issues with these levels. Small adjustments to my Warfarin dosage could be made if necessary.

Initially, I did have a bit of **difficulty keeping to my Vitamin K target**. I had always thought that I probably ate a bit too much of the Vitamin K containing foods.

However, once I started <u>tracking</u> the amount of Vitamin K that I was consuming on a daily basis I discovered that I was actually getting a lot less than I thought. On average my daily consumption was only around 50mcg, which was just 1/3 of my **target of 150mcg per day**. In an attempt to avoid eating too much Vitamin K I had actually <u>reduced my intake too much</u>!

I had fallen into the trap that so many people do when they are taking Warfarin as I had got into the habit of avoiding high Vitamin K containing foods altogether and choosing low Vitamin K alternatives.   This was probably because I knew that even just **a small amount of the high Vitamin K containing foods can significantly impact how Warfarin works** and affect my INR.

Then I had an idea.

Why not use this to my advantage?

If only very small amounts of foods like broccoli or spinach would be required to achieve my target of 150mcg of Vitamin K per day, why not use these foods in a controlled way to ensure I am hitting my daily target? If I could work out what the Vitamin K content of one brussels sprout was, for instance, I could then add the correct number of sprouts, needed to **reach my daily goal**, to whatever I was cooking or eating.

So that's what I did. I worked out the Vitamin K content of a number of small servings of foods rich in Vitamin K.

Serving	Average Weight	Approx. Vitamin K content
1 frozen **brussels sprout**	15g*	20mcg
1 fresh **broccoli** floret, raw	28g	50mcg
1 frozen **broccoli** floret	50g*	35mcg
1 cup of raw **spinach**	30g	120mcg
1 frozen **spinach** cluster	45g*	250mcg

* weight with ice glaze

I chose frozen vegetables, in the main, as these were things that I could always have in stock <u>ready to use</u> when required. The other great thing about this type of **green vegetable** is that these small amounts <u>add virtually nothing to my daily calorie total</u>!

I like to think of these as little '**doses**' of Vitamin K which I can use to keep my intake <u>consistent</u>.

So, on a daily basis, I try to keep the content of Vitamin K in the food I eat fairly moderate and <u>top up with Vitamin K 'doses' as required</u>. I find this a very simple and controlled way to ensure I am getting **the right levels of Vitamin K required for good health** without affecting my Warfarin therapy. The high Vitamin K containing foods have now become my friends again, instead of something to be avoided!

Here are a couple of examples of how this works in practice.

Example 1

I have already used 80mcg of my daily Vitamin K allowance between my breakfast, lunch and what I am having for my evening meal. I decide to steam two frozen broccoli florets and add these to my dinner to ensure that I meet my days' target.

Example 2

I have been tracking my Vitamin K intake throughout the day and between breakfast, lunch and a couple of snacks I have had 20mcg of Vitamin K. The lamb curry that I am going to cook for my evening meal is for 2 people and each serving contains 5mcg of Vitamin K. This will bring my total for the day to just 25mcg – 125mcg short of my daily target. To bring me up to the required amount for the day I decide to add 1 frozen spinach cluster to the lamb curry, adding 250mcg of Vitamin K in total which will result in an extra 125mcg per serving.

Example 3

I know I am about 50mcg short on my daily Vitamin K target so I just grab a fresh broccoli floret and munch on it raw – yum!

Anyway, getting back to my choice of diet, in addition to setting Vitamin K and Protein targets I wanted to be able to limit my calorie and fat intake and reduce my carbohydrate consumption. I started looking around for a diet that would accommodate all my requirements and allow me to achieve my goals.

I eventually decided to try the **Intermittent Fasting**, or **5:2**, diet which was first brought to the attention of the British public by the BBC Horizon programme *Eat, Fast and Live Longer* with **Dr Michael Mosley**. For anyone not familiar with this diet it basically consists of eating normally for 5 days a week and having **2 'fast' days per week** when calorie intake should be restricted to 500 calories if you are a **woman**, or restricted to 600 calories if you are a **man**. Not only does it aid weight loss but it has also been shown to be *extremely beneficial to health*.

This has to be the best, and easiest, diet I have ever been on and fits in well with all my requirements. And yes! **I have lost weight <u>and</u> my INR remains stable**.

These are some of the reasons it seems to work so well for me.

I can easily plan my protein and Vitamin K intake on both **fast** and **non-fast days**. I only need to have 2 days where I am really strict about what I eat, but these are so **simple** that it is <u>easy to stick to</u>. I know exactly what I am going to be eating on a fast day so eating 'clean' is not a problem. I can be more relaxed about my eating on the non-fast days. However, I have found that, in general, I don't require to eat that much on the non-fast days and I am more drawn to fresh, unprocessed foods. It is also so **<u>flexible</u>**. I normally have my fast days on a <u>Tuesday</u> and a <u>Thursday</u> but on weeks when I am travelling, or have other engagements, it is so easy to **swap** the days about.

So what does a fast day look like for me?

I choose to eat my 500 calories as two meals – **breakfast** and **dinner**.

I start the day with **porridge** because it is filling and nutritious and because I love it! I am able to add a few extras and still keep to **203 calories per portion**,

40g   Organic Gluten Free Porridge Oats

1 cup   Coconut Milk

½ tsp   Honey

½ tsp   Ground Cinnamon

This <u>sets me up for the day</u> and I <u>don't eat again until dinner time</u>.

One thing I struggled with initially on the 5:2 diet was getting the **right vegetables** to go with my fast day dinner time meals. A lot of the lower calories recipes I looked at contained vegetables which were rich in Vitamin K. I would have tended to have a side salad instead of vegetables before I was on Warfarin, but now this is not the best thing.   I eventually came up with two recipes I really like which **contain vegetables lower in vitamin K** (which I can add Vitamin K 'doses' to, if required).

A *Veggie Chilli* so tasty you don't miss the meat – **250 calories**

My take on *Chicken Curry* which is really delicious –
250 calories

I don't have any rice to accompany these dishes but
instead I will include a portion of spaghetti squash or
sautéed courgette spirals which **adds less than 50
calories** to my meal. You can find the recipes for all
of these in the next chapter.

So I now have two set meals which I eat alternately
on fast days. This keeps things nice and **simple**
and to **make life easier** I prepare these in bulk and
freeze single servings so I just have to pull one out of
the freezer that morning and heat through at dinner
time.

On the **other five days** of the week I am fairly **careful**
about what I eat but I am *not strict about calorie
counting*. However, to maintain consistency I do
keep track of my Vitamin K and **protein** intake to
ensure I am around my target amount. This helps to
keep my INR stable.

On my five 'normal' days I try to eat according to
some simple guidelines that I have set for myself.
I prefer to call them guidelines rather than rules as
anything too rigid makes me want to rebel! *It's a
subconscious thing.*

- I will eat only fresh, unprocessed food, wherever possible.

- I avoid gluten.

- I try and eat oily fish twice a week.

- I will only eat rice a maximum of 2 times a week.

- When I need a little treat, I have a piece of dark chocolate (preferably over 70% cocoa content).

- If I want to sweeten something I use honey or maple syrup. I try to avoid raw sugar.

- No fizzy drinks, especially diet ones.

- The only oils I use are olive oil (for eating) and coconut oil (for cooking).

- I eat from small plates and try to keep portions to around the size of my hand.

- I like to use ionised water for drinking water, tea and herbal tea.

- I choose organic ingredients where possible.

- I allow myself a day off to eat whatever I fancy from time to time – often when I have family over on a Sunday. One day here and there will not do me any harm.

Occasionally I will fall off the wagon and have a few days when I don't follow my own guidelines, <u>or even stick to my fasting</u>! We all have times when life takes over and we lose focus. How do I deal with this? Well I don't get angry with myself. I just accept I have had a '***few days off***', see it as a <u>bonus</u> and get back to my eating plan <u>without regret</u>.

The other **key to my success** is that I have taken a <u>*whole body approach*</u> to losing weight and getting healthy. By this I mean that, rather than just focussing on my **eating**, I have also used **exercise**, **meditation** and **positive thinking** to contribute towards achieving my aims.

I have a <u>twice daily workout walking my dog</u> and I do a <u>Pilates class</u> two times a week. I also try and do <u>5 minutes each day</u> on a <u>rebounder</u> as this helps to **flush out my adrenal glands** daily which in turn helps the body with its functions.

The **meditation** and **positive thinking** have been about getting my *mind into a state that will support a new way of eating*. I have spent a lot of time looking at the **<u>importance of the subconscious (unconscious) mind in managing our behaviours</u>** so when I started on this eating plan I spent a while getting my head into a good place to accept the necessary changes. I try and have only positive thoughts about food and my diet. I think about how much this eating plan is benefitting me and making me more and more healthy each day. This assists me to fully **commit to the plan** and is particularly helpful on fast days when I may start to feel a little hungry from time to time.

So what has been the outcome of this new eating plan for me?

Well, as already said, I have found this to be the **easiest diet** I have ever tried. I eat well and eat healthily and I rarely feel hungry. I have now had a number of **consistent INR readings** which are **within my desired therapeutic range**.

At the time of writing, I have managed to **lose one stone**. This didn't happen overnight, just in case you are looking for a quick fix ('quick fixes' and sudden changes are not a good idea when you are on Warfarin)! However, the weight loss has been **steady** and is **sustainable** in the long term, all while **keeping my bloods stable**. I am continuing with the eating plan and expect to achieve further slow, but steady, weight loss until I reach my goal.

More importantly I feel confident that I will be able to *maintain both my target weight and my target INR.*

This is my eating plan and it has worked really well for me. While I cannot guarantee everyone success in weight loss, or achieving a stable INR, there is no reason why you too can't succeed in reaching your own goals.

The plan is flexible enough to allow you to set your own targets and to accommodate your own specific likes and dietary needs. You may require a diet low in potassium (for your kidneys), low in cholesterol (to maintain heart health) or you may need to monitor your sugar intake (due to diabetes). This type of plan can easily be adapted to cover all of these requirements, and more. Our website, www.eatonwarfarin.com contains a number of tools to help you monitor and track your diet.

Remember, **always consult your doctor** before making any big changes to your diet. It is also important to **get your INR checked regularly** so that any fluctuations are picked up quickly and your Warfarin dosage can be adjusted, if required.

CHAPTER 7

Sample Recipes

In the previous chapter I told you about a couple of 'favourite' dinners that I eat on my 'fast' days. The recipes for these are given below. For each of these I have detailed the Vitamin K and protein content as well as providing calorie and fat totals.

Cath's Veggie Chilli (serves 4)

Delicious and extremely satisfying – you won't miss the meat! Will freeze beautifully so get organised and make a big batch!

Contains per serving

Vitamin K (µg)	- 17.5
Protein (g)	- 12.7
Calories (kcal)	- 250
Fat (g)	- 6.9

For this recipe you will need

2 carrots

3 sticks of celery

1 medium onion

1 tbsp coconut butter

2 green chillies

2 garlic cloves

6 mushrooms, sliced

2 tsp cayenne pepper

1 tsp ground cumin

1 tsp ground cinnamon

2 tbsp tomato puree

400g tinned chopped tomatoes

400g tin chickpeas

400g tin kidney beans

1 bay leaf

salt and pepper

- Finely chop the carrots, celery and onion.

- Melt the coconut butter in large pan and add the chopped vegetables.

- Add a tbsp. of water and a pinch of salt and black pepper and fry gently for 5 minutes.

- Deseed the chillies and then finely chop both the chillies and garlic. Add to the pan along with the mushrooms and stir in. Fry gently for another 5 minutes.

- Add the spices and stir to coat all the vegetables.

- Add the tomato puree, tinned tomatoes and 250ml of water and bring to the boil stirring all the time. Reduce to a simmer and cook for 20 minutes.

- Drain and rinse the chickpeas and kidney beans.

- Add the peas and beans to the pan along with a bay leaf.

- Season to taste and cook gently for a further 20 minutes until the sauce has thickened nicely.

Tips

Good served with some low fat crème fraiche but remember to add the extra calories if using!

Cath's Chicken Curry (serves 4)

I love this recipe! I pop it in the oven before walking the dog and dinner is ready on my return!

Contains per serving

Vitamin K (µg)	- 8
Protein (g)	- 24.8
Calories (kcal)	- 250
Fat (g)	- 8.5

For this recipe you will need

- **2 chicken breasts**
- **2 medium onions**
- **1 small kohlrabi (can use celeriac)**
- **1 tbsp coconut butter**
- **1 tsp cumin seeds**
- **½ tsp mustard seeds**
- **2 tsp cayenne pepper**
- **1 tsp ground cumin**
- **1 tsp ground cinnamon**
- **400g tinned chopped tomatoes**

125ml water

1 tbsp flaxseeds (optional)

2 tbsp mango chutney

50ml half fat crème fraiche

salt and pepper

- Cut the chicken breast into chunks.

- Chop the onions and cut the kohlrabi into 1cm cubes.

- Melt the coconut butter in an oven proof pan or casserole.

- Add the cumin seeds and mustard seeds and fry for 2 minutes.

- Add the onions and kohlrabi and fry for a further 5 minutes.

- Add the spices and chicken and stir for a minute until everything is coated.

- Add the tinned tomatoes and water and bring gently to the boil stirring all the time. Season to taste.

- Transfer to the oven and cook for 40 minutes at 170°C/350°F/Gas mark 4.

- 5 minutes before the cooking time is up stir in the flaxseeds (if using) and the mango chutney. Return to the oven to finish cooking.

- Remove from the oven and stir through the half fat crème fraiche.

- Serve immediately.

Tips

Freeze what you haven't used in individual portions. Great for days when you haven't got time to cook.

Spaghetti Squash

I use this as an alternative to pasta or rice. Spaghetti squash can be hard to source but well worth the effort. You don't need any fancy gadgets, it's mega easy to make and can be stored in the freezer.

Contains per serving (150g)

Vitamin K (µg)	- 1.2
Protein (g)	- 0.9
Calories (kcal)	- 46
Fat (g)	- 0.9

For this recipe you will need

1 spaghetti squash

- Preheat the oven to 200°C/400°F/Gas mark 6.

- Cut the spaghetti squash in half (this can be quite hard when the squash is raw so, alternatively, pierce the squash a few times and cook whole, doubling the cooking time).

- Scoop out the seeds with a spoon (the seeds can be kept and roasted like pumpkin seeds if you want).

- Lay both halves face down on a baking tray, place in the oven and bake for around 30 minutes (an hour if whole).

- Remove from oven and let the squash cool for about 10 minutes.

- If you cooked the squash whole, cut it in half now and carefully remove the seeds with a spoon.

- Now take each half in turn and, using a fork, scrape out the flesh. It will come away in long strands – now you can see why it is called 'spaghetti' squash!

- Serve immediately.

Tips

While perfect as an accompaniment for dishes like curry or chilli, spaghetti squash can also be eaten on its own. Serve with a little olive oil or butter and use garlic and herbs for added flavour.

If planning to freeze some, or all, of the spaghetti squash – bake the half squash in the oven for 20 minutes only, then cool and freeze. When needed, defrost, bake for a further 20 minutes and then continue as above.

Courgette Spirals (serves 1)

Another great alternative to pasta – courgettes were just born to be spiralised! You'll need a spiralizer to make these but, with such an easy, fuss free method of vegetable preparation, you will not regret the investment!

Contains per serving (150g)

Vitamin K (µg)	- 5
Protein (g)	- 2.7
Calories (kcal)	- 27
Fat (g)	- 0.6

For this recipe you will need

1 medium courgette

- Chop both ends off the courgette.

- Place the courgette in the spiralizer with the desired cutter and create spirals.

- Pat the spirals dry with a paper towel to remove excess moisture.

Eat Raw

- Courgette spirals can be eaten raw.

- They are particularly delicious used in salads with a dressing.

Boil

- Bring a large pan of water to the boil.

- Add the spirals and cook for exactly 2 minutes.

- Drain and serve immediately.

Sauté

- Heat ½ teaspoon of coconut oil in a large pan.

- Add the spirals and sauté for 3-5 minutes until tender.

- Serve immediately.

- This cooking method will add 20 calories and 2.5g of fat to each serving.

Tips

For extra flavour you can add herbs, garlic and/or chilli when sautéing the spirals.

For more great recipes along these lines go to www.eatonwarfarin.com

CHAPTER 8

Eating Out

*Keeping track of what you are eating can be hard enough when you are at home and in your own routine. Then, you go away for a week! A week of **eating out** and **unfamiliar food**! <u>Bang goes the routine and the settled INR</u>!*

This has been quite a problem for me as I often travel to London to do courses and meetings. Being away from my own fridge and not having access to my 'usual' meals makes it more difficult to ensure I am eating a balanced amount of Vitamin K and protein.

I have learned to manage this in a couple of different ways.

First of all I spent a little time getting familiar with the Vitamin K and protein content of a variety of ingredients that are in the type of dishes I would eat when out at a restaurant. This has made me far more <u>aware of what I should avoid, and what I can have instead</u>.

*Take salad, for instance. If I am ordering a salad I will ask what type of lettuce they use. If the waiter says **Cos**, or **Romaine**, lettuce (which I know is high in Vitamin K) I will ask if this could be <u>substituted</u>*

with **Rocket** or **Iceberg** lettuce which has a lower Vitamin K content. Similarly, if I have not had enough Vitamin K towards my daily target that day, I may ask for a small amount of Vitamin K rich vegetable to be <u>added</u> to my meal.

Another 'trick' that I use in moderation is having a **glass of wine**! If the particular dish I have chosen has an ingredient like **spinach**, which contains a lot of Vitamin K, I will counteract this by treating myself to a glass of wine. Put simply, as too much Vitamin K could lead to a decrease in my INR, I am <u>balancing</u> this by taking some alcohol which has the effect of increasing INR.

We are all different so what works for me may not work for someone else - always speak to your doctor about what is right for you. I think the main thing to remember is that we can still have a life on Warfarin and enjoy ourselves. The important thing is to be mindful to <u>avoid</u> **binge drinking** or making **sudden changes** to our eating patterns.

Please remember that we are all different and some of the material contained in this book relates specifically to my journey in learning to manage my diet while taking Warfarin. I am not a medical practitioner and I am not offering medical advice. There are plenty of other books available that offer a more detailed explanation of Warfarin from a medical perspective. My aim, however, has been to provide a straightforward guide that gives quick access to some of the important aspects of taking Warfarin for anyone who has been prescribed this drug. I hope other Warfarin users will find this useful.

List of Resources Used

Leaflet insert from Warfarin medication

www.nhs.uk

McCance and Widdowson's The Composition of Foods 7th Summary Edition, 2014

USDA Nutrient Database for Standard Reference Release 27

Nutescu EA, Shapiro NL, Ibrahim S, West P – Warfarin and its interactions with foods, herbs and other dietary supplements. *Expert Opin. Drug Saf. (2006) 5(3):433-451*

Biss TT, Adamson AJ, Seal CJ, Kamali F (2011). The potential impact of dietary vitamin K status on anticoagulation control in children receiving Warfarin. *Paediatric Haematology & Oncology, 28(5), 425-427. doi:10.3109/08880018.2011.562276*

Johnson MA – Influence of Vitamin K on Anticoagulant Therapy Depends on Vitamin K Status and the Source and Chemical Forms of Vitamin K. *Brief Critical Reviews March 2005: 91-100*

Bolton Smith C, Price RJG, Fenton ST, Harrington DJ, Shearer MJ – Compilation of a provisional UK database for the phylloquinone (vitamin K1) content of foods – *British Journal of Nutrition (2000), 83 389-399*

Barclay L – Vitamin K and Warfarin – *Life Extension Magazine June 2007*

Shearer MJ, Bach A, Kohlmeier M – Chemistry, Nutritional Sources, Tissue Distribution and Metabolism of Vitamin K with Special Reference to Bone Health – *The Journal of Nutrition 0022-3166/96*

Prynne CJ, Thane CW, Prentice A, Wadsworth MEJ - Intake and sources of phylloquinone (vitamin K1) in 4-year-old British children - *Public Health Nutrition (2005)*

Beatty SJ, Mehta BH, Rodis JL – Decreased Warfarin Effect After Initiation of High-Protein, Low-Carbohydrate Diets – *The Annals of Pharmacotherapy*

Tom Wan-Chih – Warfarin-Food Interactions – *Pharmacist's Letter/Prescriber's Letter May 2005 – Volume 21 – Number 210507*

Useful Links

Anticoagulation Europe (UK)

www.anticoagulationeurope.org

Arrhythmia Alliance

www.heartrhythmcharity.org.uk

Atrial Fibrillation Association

www.atrialfibrillation.org.uk

British Heart Foundation

www.bhf.org.uk

British Lung Foundation

www.blf.org.uk

Chest, Heart & Stroke – Scotland

www.chss.org.uk

Chest, Heart & Stroke – Northern Ireland

www.nichs.org.uk

Hughes Syndrome Foundation

www.hughes-syndrome.org

Lifeblood: The Thrombosis Charity

www.thrombosis-charity.org.uk

Stroke Association

www.stroke.org.uk

Index